LYMPHOLOGY

"DON'T WAIT TILL YOU'RE DISEASED"

100 CASE STUDIES

Revitalize, Rejuvenate, And Restore Cellular Regeneration
Lymphology Australia - Reversing The Impossible

BY MICHELLE J RICHARDSON

LYMPHOLOGIST

First published 2025

A self published title
Designed and produced by Adala Publishing
www.adalapublishing.com.au

A catalogue record for this
book is available from the
National Library of Australia

NATIONAL
LIBRARY
OF AUSTRALIA

ISBN: 978-1-7640649-0-3 (Print)
ISBN: 978-1-7640649-1-0 (eBook)

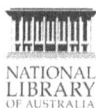

Contents

Dedication

ONCE, THERE LIVED A man whose wealth was not measured in gold but in abundant knowledge and the art of giving. He walked through life with a rare presence—his vision and thoughts ever focused on a single, profound goal: healing the world. He foresaw a future teetering on the edge of catastrophe, a grim era where disease would claim one in three lives, leaving families shattered and nations in mourning. His predictions, made in 1990, seemed almost prophetic, for here we are today, struggling to hold onto life as parents, children, friends, and colleagues succumb before our eyes.

This man, C. Samuel West, was more than a healer. He was a beacon of honor, hope, and the belief in humanity's ability to transform its destiny. With an unyielding determination, he dedicated himself to unveiling a truth that could change the course of history: the human body holds within it the power to heal itself, and the key lies in understanding the intricate, life-giving system of Lymphology.

Samuel's vision was not merely one of survival but of thriving—of creating a world where disease no longer held dominion, where education empowered individuals to take charge of their health, and where the art of self-healing became a birthright. He knew that if he did nothing, the world would spiral into an era of destruction.

But Samuel proved that one man's vision could become the blueprint for a healthier, more resilient world with every step he took, every person he taught, and every life he touched.

This was the journey of a man who defied the relentless currents of illness and despair, forging a path of healing and transformation that continues to inspire the world. His unwavering dedication left a legacy of renewed hope for his time and countless generations to follow. Today, his son, Karl West, carries the torch, boldly advancing the mission his father began—empowering lives and reshaping the future of health.

These were my teachings, my truth, and my gift to the world...

Foreword
By Professor Karl West

IMAGINE PURCHASING A HIGH-PERFORMANCE automobile. Besides having no defects in the production of that car, would you also expect to receive a copy of the owner's manual so you can care for it well? Yes, you would. You would want to know how to care for it best, right?

Yet, how much more crucial might it be to have a manual for caring for your body? Would you believe that at least 50% of the actual science of healing pertains to the role of your lymphatic system?

My name is Karl J. West, and my father, Dr. C. Samuel West, gave up his academic career, including retirement, after he researched life-saving discoveries involving the lymphatic system. In order to teach people how to heal their own bodies, to save lives, and to prevent unnecessary suffering, my father dedicated the remainder of his life to teaching the public about the discoveries of the vital role of the lymphatic system in maintaining proper circulation and how to make this system work more effectively for you. He wrote a book called *The Golden Seven Plus One,* an Introduction to the Science of Lymphology, teaching a method he called the Art of Lymphasizing.

I recently read Michelle Richardson's book, *100 Case Studies*, which provides remarkable insights and practical examples in lymphology. It is an invaluable resource highlighting the real-world applications of lymphatic treatments and their benefits. By combining our knowledge and experiences, we can contribute positively to this field and explore new ways to help those in need. Thank you for considering my message, and congratulations on your wise decision to purchase her book.

Introduction

I AM A GUIDE, gifted with a deep understanding of innate intelligence. This gift allows me to illuminate the truth within and around others, helping them see the unseen, heal their wounds, and reclaim their lives.

This book is a profound journey into the essence of healing, where intuition intertwines with wisdom. It tells the story of one woman's extraordinary ability to transform lives, turning pain into peace and suffering into unshakable strength.

MY STORY IN SHORT...

School years

My schooling was plagued by social conflict. I was the only one who sat next to the only overweight kid back in the seventies, who was ostracized and taunted by everyone else.

Her unwashed clothes carried a pungent, sour odor that clung to the air around her, making others wrinkle their noses and keep their distance, as if she were a walking contagion. The other kids whispered cruelly behind her back, their judgement as sharp as their avoidance. Yet, despite her ostracization, I couldn't help but feel an inexplicable pull toward her. Maybe it was the way her downcast eyes mirrored a loneliness I recognized all too well, or perhaps it was a budding empathy, born from my own struggles with being different.

Together, we were labeled as weirdos and bullied relentlessly. My triplet sisters hated it for two reasons: they despised seeing me bullied, and they couldn't understand why I chose to sit next to the most disliked kid in school, but that was my reality as a child: navigating a world that lacked compassion, and it was confusing.

As a child, I was very quiet. It wasn't until my much later years that I started to find my voice. Diagnosed with dyslexia at a young age, I struggled to express myself, and the constant nagging from my parents to speak up and speak properly only added to my frustration. I couldn't understand why I felt so different, and the confusion and shame I carried, over time, turned into bitterness. This bitterness festered inside me, fueling anger and aggression. It became my coping mechanism, a shield that protected me from the hurt of not being understood. My childhood was a swirl of frustration, feeling misunderstood and isolated. These feelings affect so many young people today.

I frequently caught myself having conversations with myself, a habit that sometimes felt downright crazy, yet there was always a response. The voice behind these answers remained a mystery, but it was always there. The responses felt like a roller coaster ride— sometimes loud and forceful, other times soft and gentle. They ranged from words of encouragement and affirmation to feelings of unworthiness, caution, and even moments of pure joy. Nothing made sense, but I just followed the norm. My dream was to be a superhero, a childhood dream of creating change for others. Why I had a dream like this, I do not know. Growing up watching super-hero TV shows in the late seventies—Wonder Woman, Six Million

Dollar Man—to share a few. I wanted to be like them, to destroy evil and make good. It was so exciting to me.

I look at my life now and reflect on how little belief I once had in myself. The transformation I've experienced is nothing short of extraordinary. Despite the challenges and circumstances I faced, I never let them stop me from pursuing my dream of making a meaningful difference in the lives of many.

Looking back, I realize that every experience I've had has shaped me into the person I am today. The journey was never easy, and I often questioned why I had to face such challenges. But instead of falling into a victim mindset, I held onto a deeper vision—a vision of creating a space where people could learn to heal from their pain and suffering. While I didn't know exactly what that would look like at the time, I trusted that it was my purpose, and I kept moving forward.

After much learning, I started my business in the inner eastern suburbs of Melbourne in 2019. I had just returned from the USA and had joined a Lymphology practice to start applying my new skills as a lymphologist, specializing in lymphatic drainage. Then, the news of a global pandemic broke, and the world was shaken. Businesses shut down, and people were terrified, too afraid to step outside their doors. It felt completely insane to me as I had learned without a doubt—in fact my belief is so strong—that you can heal yourself from anything. Your built-in doctor is your immune system. If you make it you can reverse it.

My young years

In a time long ago, a young girl harbored a vision of healing the world, driven by an unshakable desire to create a lasting, transformative impact on the lives of countless souls. It was crazy to have such a vision and everyone thought I was nuts.

Just like everyone else, life felt like a never-ending cycle of chaos. Being a mother, a wife, a people-pleaser with a business to run, I had so much to learn to create my vision. I had two wonderful children, a girl and a boy, both grown up now with their own lives. I thought I would never reach my dreams. The years rolled on and I was always putting others first and my dreams came second. As I reflect on my life now, I'm humbled by how little belief I once had in myself. The journey I've taken feels nothing short of extraordinary. Despite the challenges and hardships that once seemed insurmountable, I refused to let them define me or deter me from following my dream—to make a meaningful and lasting difference in the lives of others.

As a mother, my days were a whirlwind of responsibilities—school pick-ups, cheering at sporting games, and working as a personal trainer before and after hours. No matter how hectic things became, I always made time for my children and family. My schedule was filled with washing endless loads of laundry, preparing healthy meals, maintaining a large house and its gardens, and striving to be a devoted wife. I constantly juggled these tasks while trying to meet everyone's expectations. "Yes, no worries, I can do that," I'd often say, even when I felt utterly overwhelmed and exhausted. Despite the chaos, I truly loved my life and the roles I played within it.

There were moments when I would speak to God—not out of religious devotion, but out of a deep belief in a higher power that placed us here for a purpose. Running became my sanctuary, the place where I could quiet the noise in my mind and hear whispers of wisdom. Mile after mile, my thoughts would flow freely, unburdened, as if the answers I sought were carried on the wind.

Running wasn't just an escape; it was my passion, my anchor. I poured myself into exercise, not just for the love of it, but because it connected me to a greater mission—changing lives. Through my personal training business, I discovered the profound joy of transforming others, helping them find strength they never thought possible.

My thirst for knowledge was insatiable. I became certified as a Pilates instructor and yoga teacher, dove into emotional intelligence, completed a basic nutrition course, and trained as a life coach. I immersed myself in countless hours of self-study, devouring lectures, attending seminars, and learning from experts in their fields.

By 2016, I added another dimension to my life's work—I trained to host my own radio show, *Pay It Forward*. Focused on intergenerational health, the show allowed me to connect with global experts and share their insights with my local community. For three incredible years, I used the airwaves to spark conversations and inspire change.

Then life shifted. My sister, Julie, fell gravely ill, and she needed me. Without hesitation, I stepped away to be by her side, knowing that some callings in life are greater than others.

We were three—triplets—born in the sixties, a surprise bundle that turned life upside down for our parents. Mum was overwhelmed, and Dad embodied the authoritarian father of the era: "Do as I say, or else." His strict demeanor unsettled Julie the most, cutting straight to her core.

Childhood shapes us in ways we often don't realize, molded by what we see, hear, and experience. Growing up in the seventies felt, at first glance, carefree and idyllic—simple days filled with innocence. But beneath the surface, life was anything but easy. Mum and

Dad grappled with the immense challenge of raising three unexpected babies alongside our two older brothers.

Life was a paradox: tough in ways we didn't fully understand, yet free of the complications we'd face as adults.

We didn't rely on doctors back then, and even now, at 58 years old, I haven't seen a doctor since I gave birth to my daughter 32 years ago, no tests, nothing. I hold an unwavering belief in the body's innate ability to heal itself. Throughout my life, I've absorbed a wealth of knowledge, but discovering the art of Lymphology and Wolfe Non-Surgical techniques was transformative. It was the pivotal moment that unlocked the true essence of healing—the missing key, the final piece of the puzzle, the holy grail of health. The beauty of this discovery is that anyone can learn it, empowering themselves and others to reclaim their health naturally.

PART 1

A thriving business
Fitness and friendship

I LOVED CHALLENGING MY clients, seeing them have fun, and encouraging them to step out of their comfort zones. Watching friendships blossom in both group and one-on-one classes was incredibly rewarding. Before I knew it, I had a thriving full-time business running from home.

Managing an indoor and outdoor gym in winter had its challenges, especially braving the cold. But there was an undeniable magic in those moments under the night sky—pushing through a bench press while watching the stars shimmer above, steam rising from our bodies into the crisp, frosty air. I was in peak form back then, leading a variety of classes: Pilates, boxing, cycling, circuit training, 8-week transformation programs, post- and pre-natal fitness, and specialized classes for older adults. The energy was electric, the business thriving, and clients kept coming back, hungry for more. It was a time of unstoppable momentum and transformation—for me and everyone I coached.

Every class was a blend of hard work and camaraderie. The energy was palpable whether we were punching bags in a boxing class or stretching muscles in a Pilates session. Regardless of age or fitness level, each client was part of a supportive community that thrived on encouragement and mutual respect. It wasn't just about physical fitness but also mental and emotional well-being.

The 8-week challenge programs were particularly popular. Clients loved setting goals and working towards them, motivated by the progress they saw in themselves and their peers. The sense of accomplishment at the end of each challenge was immense, and the transformations were often astounding. Watching someone go from doubting their abilities to smashing their goals was one of the most fulfilling aspects of my work.

Post- and pre-natal classes were another unique aspect of my business. Helping new and expectant mothers stay fit and healthy was a privilege. These classes provided a space for women to connect and share their experiences, creating a supportive network beyond the gym.

The older adults' classes were equally rewarding. Many of my clients initially hesitated to join, worried about their fitness levels or existing health conditions. But once they started, they quickly discovered that age was no barrier to enjoying exercise and reaping its benefits.

During those years, my business wasn't just about fitness; it was about creating a community where people felt supported, challenged, and inspired, could escape everyday life's stresses, and could focus on their well-being. It was a time of growth for my clients and me, as I learned as much from them as they did from me. But inside I wasn't happy.

Imagine this: life can be brutally unforgiving. My marriage shattered, leaving me divorced and alone once again. My business lost its direction and eventually closed down. Forced to sell my home,

I moved into a rented house, clinging to the hope of rebuilding my life at 47 years old.

But then, the unthinkable happened—my world collapsed even further. Julie, my beloved triplet sister, faced a devastating return of her cancer, this time more aggressive and relentless. It felt like the universe had unleashed a storm, leaving me grasping at pieces of a life that seemed to be slipping through my fingers. Where next? Julie had to get better and I had the knowledge. Off to the USA with Julie to find more answers.

Growing up Michelle

ONE SEEMINGLY ORDINARY AFTERNOON at 5 pm, my phone rang as I prepared to start my class. It was my sister, Julie. Her voice trembled as she delivered the news: "Dad has taken a turn for the worse." The weight of her words hit me like a freight train. I rushed to the hospital, and as I walked through those sterile halls, I felt my legs give way, collapsing onto the cold, tiled floor. My world stood still, the bustling sounds of the hospital fading into a distant murmur.

I was forced to confront a reality I had long avoided in that crisis. At 42 years old, I had to decide solely for myself. For years, I had relied on my husband for answers, convinced that my judgments were never good enough. I doubted my ability to make the right choices, always seeking validation from others. But this situation was different. It was about my father, the man I loved and adored.

When I was growing up, Dad was a strict figure, he ruled our household with an iron fist. He embodied the societal belief that men held the power and could do whatever they wanted. Despite his harshness, a part of me profoundly respected and cherished him. His background was a stark contrast to my own life. Dad came from a family of significant wealth—the first Richardson to own a car in the 1920s, an ice chest refrigerator, and a home staffed with maids. He enjoyed a life of luxury that seemed almost mythical to me.

As I sat in the hospital, memories of my father flooded my mind. I remembered the stories he told about his childhood, the grandeur of his family's estate, and the expectations that came with such privilege. I realized that his strictness was shaped by the pressures and standards of his upbringing. Despite the opulence of his youth, he faced his own set of challenges and responsibilities, ones that I was only beginning to understand.

In the quiet moments between the beeping of hospital machines and the hurried footsteps of nurses, I felt a profound shift within myself. I needed to let go of the past—the weight of expectations, the fear of making wrong choices, and the reliance on others for validation. This decision was mine to make. My father's condition was a catalyst for my transformation.

I resolved to be there for him, not just as a daughter but as a person reclaiming her strength and independence. The journey ahead was uncertain, but I felt a sense of clarity and purpose for the first time in my life. It was a turning point, not just in my relationship with my father, but with myself.

But with my grief of losing my dad, I had no words.

I sat quietly with Dad, keeping the night watch at the hospital. He had been there for four weeks. Eventually, my sister Julie and I found the courage to tell him it was okay to let go. Julie and I were very spiritual, not religiously, but in the belief that something else was out there. What it was, I didn't know, but it fascinated me. This electricity ran through me, even as a young child.

I remembered how Mom took us to church, and I watched people silently sit there. I always wondered why Mom wanted to hear someone talk about a book that meant nothing to me. Reflecting on our upbringing, I realized how hard Mom had it—an alcoholic who yelled and screamed late into the night, often asleep on the couch by mid-morning after a bottle of sherry. Perhaps the church was her lonely sanctuary, a place that felt safe with God. I'll never know because Mom never discusses those days with us, leaving so many secrets locked away.

In the hospital, Dad became a pin cushion for drugs as doctors struggled to diagnose his condition. It seemed like Dad had just given up—his time was up, Dad was 82. He no longer enjoyed life, his eyesight was failing and his body hurt. What was there to live for? During our conversations, I saw the fear of dying in his eyes, but I also saw a side of him I didn't know—a caring, warm man who loved his daughters. It's funny how men mellow with age, whether from wisdom or the passage of time.

We talked for hours, and during our last conversation, Dad told me, "Follow your dreams. Don't leave this planet without fulfilling your life's purpose." His words shocked me. My whole family thought I was foolish, believing life was nothing but "yes sir, no sir." Hearing this from Dad was a revelation.

When Dad was moved to the ICU, his condition had worsened. Inflammation and fluid around his lungs indicated he was shutting down. The chief of staff said it was only a matter of time. We called the family together to discuss the options. If we turned off the oxygen, Dad faced two outcomes: becoming a vegetable in a nursing home or passing on. Julie and I discussed Dad's need to let go, and we whispered in his ear, "Dad, it's time to go. We will look after Mom, and everything will be okay."

In response, Dad removed his oxygen mask and spoke words of wisdom and heart. He said goodbye to the family. Everyone was stunned—just minutes earlier, his oxygen levels were critically low.

The chief of the ICU watched this miraculous moment, as did my brother and another sister. I held Mom tightly, helping her stay calm and peaceful.

Dad raised his hand to his brother Bill and said, "Bill, I am coming." And then Dad left. The silence that followed was eerie. Julie stood there, holding the space for Dad. I didn't understand what that meant, but we eventually left. This experience changed my life forever. I had never said goodbye to anyone before. My head spun with memories of my marriage. During those four weeks, my husband only came to see Dad once. I felt the bullshit start to surface, my anger at life building up. The last 20 years were ready to spill over.

Unlikely hero

AS A CHILD, LONELINESS was my constant companion. I had no friends. My marriage years were no different—I still felt very isolated. What was it about me that drove people away? Was I so strange, so unworthy, that no-one ever stayed? I was a loner, a shadow lingering on the edges of every room.

I was an angry little girl trapped in a world that didn't understand me. My voice was broken, my words fumbled, and my courage was non-existent. Growing up as a triplet was supposed to mean built-in allies, a sisterhood of equals—but not for me. My sisters were the "it girls," radiating confidence and charm. I was the odd one out, the burden they had to endure.

Even at birth, I was last. Two older brothers had learned to fend for themselves, and I, the weakest link, came home from the hospital after everyone else. My entire childhood seemed to mirror that start—I was always coming last.

As triplets, we were inseparable in the eyes of others, yet within that trio, I felt like an intruder. My sisters tolerated my presence, but I was the tagalong no-one wanted. Their resentment was unspoken but clear, and I could feel it with every sigh and side glance.

Julie was the toughest. She was the first to leave school, the first to have a boyfriend, the first to talk back to Dad, the first to drink alcohol and smoke, and the first to climb out the window to meet friends at the local park. Meanwhile, I sat at home, as scared as a mouse, not speaking. Every time I opened my mouth, I was told to shut up. So, I did.

Julie's journey took a devastating turn when she was diagnosed with breast cancer in 2016, at just forty-seven years old. Her life had always been a battlefield. As a child, she grappled with a deep belief that Mum didn't love her—a wound that festered and shaped her adulthood. Beneath Julie's bold and defiant exterior lay a reservoir of pain, a raw and aching truth that I only began to grasp in the later chapters of her life.

During her long and grueling battle with breast cancer, Julie poured her soul into her diary. Within its pages, she revealed a truth that left me breathless—she had struggled more deeply than I ever imagined, even more than I had during my own tumultuous childhood. Julie, the sister I always saw as fearless and unwavering, the one who faced the world with unshakable strength while I hid in the shadows, had carried a hidden weight of insecurities and pain. Her words shattered the image I had of her, exposing a side I never knew—a tender, vulnerable soul who had been quietly hurting all along.

Reading her letter was like unlocking a door I never knew existed. In her words, I found a reflection of my own hidden pain. Despite our differences, we shared a common thread—a longing to be understood, a yearning for love that always seemed out of reach. Her letter wasn't just ink on paper; it was a bridge, a fragile but honest glimpse into her soul. It shattered the tough image I had of her and revealed someone fighting battles I had never imagined. In that moment, I didn't just see her as my sister; I saw her as a fellow traveler, navigating the same lonely roads in her own way.

Her words lingered with me, making me confront my own life. I thought about the walls I had built around myself, the solitude I had learned to embrace because it felt safer than rejection. Perhaps we weren't so different after all—two loners seeking something intangible, something we couldn't quite name.

As a teenager, I drifted through those years feeling utterly alone. School ended, and with it, any semblance of connection. My sisters were busy with their full-time jobs and boyfriends, living lives that seemed miles away from mine. Mum drowned her days in alcohol, and Dad's anger filled whatever space was left. My brothers had all left home by then, leaving the house eerily empty, like a shell of what it might have been.

Life has a way of weaving its tapestry with unexpected threads. I discovered a profound purpose in helping others, working hand in hand with a physiotherapist as an aide. Earning my certificate as an Allied Health Assistant felt like grasping a lifeline in a turbulent sea. Relief washed over me when I learned there was no exam to face—I was certain I'd never succeed at one. Yet, despite my doubts, a flicker of pride ignited deep within me. For the first time, I felt like I was forging something meaningful—not just for others, but for my own sense of worth and identity.

People are drawn to me in ways I can't entirely explain, as if they sense an unspoken connection, a warmth that emanates from deep within my soul. My heart swelled with every encounter, every opportunity to touch someone's life in a way that mattered. At seventeen, I embarked on my first real job at a nursing home, working alongside an extraordinary physiotherapist named Judy Shergold. Judy was unlike anyone I'd ever met—an older woman with an almost ethereal presence, whose hands seemed to carry the very essence of healing. She became my mentor, and taught me how to use touch as a language of restoration and hope.

The first time I placed my hands on someone, I felt a startling heat radiate from my palms—a warmth so vivid it seemed alive. It wasn't just physical; it was an energy that stirred something deep within me. Soon, I began to feel and perceive things I couldn't explain—subtle cues from their bodies, whispers of what they needed. This was the beginning of my journey into a world where my innate abilities would reveal themselves as a gift to bring transformation and renewal.

Today, I dedicate hours each week to helping people reclaim their lives. I guide them back to strength and independence, teaching them to walk again, to hold their loved ones, and to rediscover the simple yet profound joys of everyday life. Each step they take, each moment of regained movement, feels like witnessing a miracle—a miracle I've had the privilege to facilitate. For me, this isn't just work; it is a sacred calling, a reminder of the resilience hidden in the human spirit.

Despite the challenges and emotional weight of my work, I found immense beauty in the moments of connection it brought. Each day unfolded like a tapestry woven with stories of triumph and perseverance. I spent countless hours sitting with frail, elderly patients, holding their hands as they faced the twilight of their lives. For many, I was their sole source of comfort, the only voice in a world that had fallen silent around them. Their hands, often cold and trembling, gripped mine with a strength born of desperation and trust.

In those quiet moments, time seemed to pause. Their stories spilled out—tales of love and loss, regret and hope—and I listened with my whole being. I became their lifeline, their anchor in an ocean of uncertainty. As I sat with them, I realized that this work was not just about healing the body but about mending unseen fractures in the heart and soul.

Each life I touched left an imprint on mine. I carried their courage and pain with me, woven into the fabric of who I was becoming. It was as though my hands weren't just my own—they carried the stories, the struggles, and the triumphs of all those I had the honor to serve.

It's strange how life unfolds. We often feel we have no control over it, yet somehow, we navigate through it. My work became more than a job; it reflected my journey. I found a sense of purpose and connection in helping others, something I had longed for my entire young life.

There were moments when I looked into a patient's eyes and saw a reflection of my loneliness and fears. But in those moments of shared vulnerability, I also found strength. I realized that my experiences, struggles, and isolation had prepared me to be there for others in their time of need. It was as if my entire life had led me to this point.

I remember one patient, Mrs Joy Anderson, who had suffered a stroke. Joy was unable to speak or move her right side. The first time I met her, I could see the fear and frustration in her eyes. I spent hours with her, gently encouraging her to try, reassuring her that failing was okay, and celebrating every small victory with her. Over time, she began to regain some movement in her hand. The day Joy managed to grip my hand and squeeze it lightly was a day of triumph for both of us. In 1990, I was about to embark on one of the most exciting moments of my life—getting married—and I couldn't wait to ask Joy to join me at my wedding! Joy shared with me that she would walk with me, with the deepest of love, and her dream would come true.

In those moments, I understood that my work was more than physical rehabilitation. It was about restoring dignity and hope, being a source of comfort and strength when someone felt vulnerable, and showing that, even in our weakest moments, we are not alone.

As I sat with each person holding their hand, I realized that I was not just helping them heal; they were helping me heal, too. They taught me the power of resilience, the importance of compassion, and the beauty of human connection. Through them, I found my voice, strength, and courage, I felt peace with every one of my clients.

At work, I was someone else entirely—a force to be reckoned with. I wasn't judged or dismissed; I was respected. People looked up to me. I was *Michelle*, a person of value and purpose. But at home, I shrank into the shadows. I was the girl who couldn't speak, who couldn't write, who was destined to fail—at least, that's how my family saw me. No-one knew of my achievements, no-one cared to ask, and no-one thought it mattered. That disconnect, that invisibility, had become my normal. My life at home was a world where dreams didn't exist, and accomplishments were unacknowledged whispers in the void.

As a teenager in the dynamic, colorful eighties, life brimmed with boundless promise. Dad's relentless dedication ensured we had the privilege of attending private school, though my sister Julie took a different route, leaving after ninth grade—a time when further education wasn't a pressing priority. Despite our shared beginnings,

Julie rose to remarkable heights, achieving the extraordinary dis-
tinction of becoming the youngest manager at Susan's fashion store
in the bustling city by the age of just 17. Her accomplishments left
me awestruck. Julie embodied everything I yearned for—elegant
clothes, financial freedom, and dazzling success.

Burning with envy, I couldn't resist raiding Julie's closet, unearth-
ing her hidden treasures and draping myself in her charm—always
in secret. She loathed my invasions and would never grant permission; the mere thought of her icy rejection was enough to paralyze
me. Still, my longing to be her—to *feel* like her—drove me to steal
moments that weren't mine. I craved her effortless confidence, her
magnetic presence at parties, and her circle of admirers. But every
time I gazed at my reflection, our striking resemblance felt like a
cruel joke, highlighting the chasm between her radiant spirit and
my fractured self.

2021 time of change

CHRIS WAS MY HAIRDRESSER of thirty years. Once you find a great hairdresser, you stick with them. Chris had a spare room at the back of his shop, and he offered to share it with me, allowing me to rent a room for my lymphology and lymphatic drainage massage practice. No-one had heard of lymphology before, and being away from the city, I wondered if I would attract a new clientele, especially since I had left a massive client base back in the city. I questioned whether they would travel to the hills for my services.

I was now renting a private place and a separate rental for my business. I wondered if it was too much to handle and if I was brave enough to start again. I had no choice but to move forward because I loved my work. It wasn't just work; it was a calling to teach people how to heal. I've never relied on a GP, never faced serious illness, and the worst I've experienced is a fleeting runny nose. Every single day, my body and spirit rise as unstoppable forces were healing and protecting me without my command. This unshakable trust in my body's innate power is proof of the extraordinary potential we all possess to thrive.

I often wonder why I've always possessed this innate ability to believe in the body's power to heal itself. It's been 32 years since I last visited a doctor—when I gave birth to my daughter. Since then,

I haven't been sick. My unwavering faith in my body's resilience and natural processes has guided me through life, allowing me to remain healthy and strong. With this belief I push on to continue my divine path.

At the beginning of 2022, I was fortunate that a few clients traveled to see me. I started a marketing campaign to rebuild the business. Life was hard after Covid-19, and I trusted my creator to build a strong belief that this was it.

After 12 months of building a thriving client base, my business was flourishing, and it was time to take a bold step forward—expanding into a larger space and reaching new heights. One day, during a conversation with my hairdresser Chris, fate intervened. Chris introduced me to Judy, who unexpectedly entered my life and brought a spark of new opportunities.

PART 2
CASE STUDIES

**FROM THE START OF THIS JOURNEY
1 TO 100**

1 JUDY

Judy was an extraordinary older lady with a spark that could light up the dullest room. Her vivacious energy and zest for life belied her years, and she carried herself with a grace that drew people in. One day, Judy confided in me about her nagging back issues, her voice tinged with a mix of hope and curiosity. I instinctively knew I could help her, and we wasted no time.

The very next day, Judy found herself nestled in the soothing embrace of the energy bed, experiencing a gentle lymphatic drainage massage paired with energy healing. Her body seemed to respond with gratitude, and her spirit radiated an undeniable vitality.

As I worked with Judy, a sudden thought struck me like a revelation. Why not ask her to join me in the office? Her sharp sense of justice, coupled with her boundless kindness, left an indelible impression on me. At 79, Judy was not only a perfect fit but an inspiration—a testament to how life continues to thrive when we nurture it.

Judy's story is one of resilience, purpose, and the magic of embracing the unexpected...

I have known Michelle for the past few years and have seen the vast difference in the clients she has helped. I decided to incorporate her teachings and listen to her suggestions about the importance of her research.

All the research on diabetes, blood pressure, and cholesterol tablets is found to have many harmful side effects on people. Being much older, I had never thought to query what the doctors were telling me, and up until this point, I had never thought to do any research on this sort of thing. I believed [what the doctors were saying must be right; the doctor knows best] it's what I was always taught.

Eighteen months ago, I was prescribed by western doctors. I needed to be on several medications, they were telling me if I didn't take them I would possibly die. GREAT SCARE TACTIC! The only results I found from the medications were extra weight gain, and no matter what I ate or didn't eat, I kept putting it on.

I decided that I would go off all medications but keep them just in case and see what would happen without them. Before going off those pills, I weighed 63 kg, way over what I should have been for my overall size. I found that just walking to the shops, I was totally out of breath and had to stop before continuing on my way, which was quite distressing for me as I had always been so fit. I could only put it down to the weight gain.

I am now 80 years old, and since stopping taking these drugs, which were the cause of the weight gain, I lost 12 kg, and I am back to me of years ago and feeling the best ever.

Apart from the drugs, the main thing I stopped consuming was sugar in anything, and as always, making sure that what I eat is homemade, NOT supermarket packaged foods or take-aways. Fresh is BEST.

I'm not suggesting that everyone do what I have done, but I strongly recommend that everyone research the medications they are given and decide if they are right for them. Also, ask the doctor many questions about their diagnosis.

Judy had been hesitant about continuing her medication, even though she knew it was causing her to gain weight without providing any real benefits. One day, she asked me for help to get off the medication, and I agreed without hesitation. I assured her we would monitor her blood pressure daily and incorporate some exercise, starting with just 10 minutes on the stationary bike. We would take it step by step from there. On the first day, we did the exercise together. I asked Judy how she felt, and she responded enthusiastically, "Great!" I took her weight and measurements to ensure she wasn't losing muscle mass, which is crucial for maintaining bone density. Within a week, Judy felt fantastic, and the weight started falling as the weeks passed. Judy's progress was remarkable. She continued to lose weight steadily and noticed significant improvements in her overall health and energy levels. Her blood pressure stabilized, and she felt more vibrant and alive than in years.

Before long, Judy reached her goal weight. Her transformation was nothing short of inspirational. Every time someone new walks into the clinic, they are greeted with Judy's beaming smile and her story of perseverance and success. She is a picture of health, radiating confidence and vitality, and serves as a living testament to the power of determination and a well-structured plan.

Judy's journey has become a beacon of hope for many others. With proper support and commitment, she achieved her health goals. Her story inspires those who visit the clinic, showing them they can also take control of their health and transform their lives.

2   SUE

Once, there was a remarkable woman who needed my help. A good friend of mine had a friend, Sue, who was in severe pain due to shingles. Sue was a farm lady who loved riding horses and led a busy life on her farm with her long-term husband. Sue had no children and found herself struggling, ill, and alone. Sue had spent the last four weeks in the hospital, but her condition hadn't improved. This happened four years before I discovered Lymphology. At the time, I was practicing Flame Tree, a personal development healing system that involves mapping out the body's innate intelligence and using various techniques to reverse illness and disease.

Sue arrived and sat on the clinic table, ready to explain her ailments. I reassured her, saying, "No need to tell me. Your innate intelligence will guide me." I planned to map out the situation with my tendon response and proceed. Sue was skeptical, and I was nervous, wondering if this would even work. But I believed in my teacher and the program, having witnessed miracles through this therapy.

I guided Sue through deep breathing exercises, helping her relax into peace and calm. Then, we began uncovering what was wrong with her emotionally, spiritually, and physically. It was a process of elimination, getting down to the cellular level. We discovered Sue was suffering from shingles and that a red jacket was connected to her hallway closet.

Sue was puzzled. "What does a red jacket have to do with my illness?" she asked.

"It seems you have an emotional block related to this jacket," I explained. "It belonged to your mother, and while you don't want to throw it out, you also hate it."

This unresolved emotional stress was wreaking havoc on her large intestine, causing the infection to grow out of control and creating painful, disabling inflammation. Other issues surfaced as we worked through each frequency level around her body.

After employing various techniques to clear the energy and unblock the charges and triggers causing Sue's sickness, her body felt light and at peace at the end of the session. We identified the shingles and other heavy metals in her body. Additionally, the red jacket symbolized a strained relationship with her mother, filled with bitterness and loneliness, which caused immense stress. This emotional turmoil weakened Sue's immune system, making her incapable of fighting the infection.

Sue was astonished by my insights. "How did you know all this?" she asked.

"I didn't," I replied. "Your body and spirit told me."

"Wow, how do you do that?" Sue wondered.

"I don't know, but it's working," I said.

Sue went home, struggling to explain the experience to her husband, but she felt alive again. Within a few days, her energy began to return. She was back to riding her horse after six months of being unable to, despite her doctors saying she would never ride again at her age, which was her early 60s. Sue also got rid of her red jacket. Sue returned a few more times for follow-up sessions and has remained healthy.

A journey of healing

I hadn't seen Sue for a few years, but she suddenly reappeared in my life. As she entered the reception area of my clinic, I could hear her talking, her voice almost breaking with stress and grief.

I welcomed Sue with open arms, and she immediately poured out her emotions, a whirlwind of grief and sadness. Her sister had passed away only six months ago, her long-time companion, her horse, had just died, and her husband of 40 years had come home after two brain surgeries, hoping for the best. Sue had been in survival mode, traveling to see her sick sister in the country, dealing with doctors and specialist visits, acting as the taxi driver, and waiting for results, all while not knowing the outcomes. It was emotionally draining for Sue. Despite not being young, she had to keep going, but the toll was evident. She was losing weight, not eating, not sleeping, and utterly exhausted.

Sue lay down on the SOQI bed and immediately felt calm and relaxed. I asked if she would like to grieve for her sister and say goodbye, as she hadn't had the time to mourn any of her losses until now, three months later. I created a space for her to open up, bring her sister forward, speak to her, release her emotions, and lovingly say goodbye. This process allowed Sue to return to peace and harmony.

After just one hour, Sue left feeling amazing, with a lightness of freedom and newfound joy. Even though Sue was still caring for her husband, who was on the mend, she had reclaimed a sense of peace and balance. Still, Sue comes back to check on me to ensure I am okay. Seeing her every few weeks is a joy.

3   ALBERT

Albert walked into my clinic on a Friday afternoon, looking utterly exhausted, broken, and hopeless. The weight of his struggles dulled his once vibrant eyes. Albert sat and began to chat about his life, recounting his recent endeavors. Albert wasn't quite sure what he had stepped into; his daughter had suggested he find someone proficient in lymphatic drainage to help clear the waste from his system. Knowing a little more, he started sharing his story with Judy and me.

Several weeks ago, Albert began feeling perpetually fatigued and flat. Despite this, he continued working as a concreter—a grueling job for anyone, let alone a 72-year-old. His resilience was admirable, but the toll on his body was evident. His skin appeared dehydrated, his posture slumped forward, and he complained of severe pain around his waistline. Eating had become a challenge, though Albert still had a solid build.

Albert's condition was concerning. His physical symptoms and the look of despair in his eyes told a story of a man struggling against the relentless wear and tear of his labor-intensive job. As he spoke, it became clear that his body was crying out for relief, and it was our mission to provide him with the healing Albert so desperately needed.

A few months ago, Albert's family suggested he get tested for stage 4 inflammation of his prostate. He was taken aback, as this seemed unrelated to the fatigue and discomfort he was experiencing. Nonetheless, he went for the test, and sure enough, he was diagnosed with stage 4 inflammation. As a Lymphologist, I knew this indicated a significant waste buildup in his body.

Albert's PSA (Prostate-Specific Antigen) test results were alarmingly high. This revelation terrified him, even though he didn't fully understand the implications. PSA is an enzyme released in the prostate, and its abnormally high concentration in the blood is often associated with prostate cancer (waste in the blood). An enzyme is a substance that acts as a catalyst in living organisms, regulating the rate of chemical reactions without being altered. These reactions are vital for biological processes, most of which enzymes control.

Albert's diagnosis indicated a severe imbalance in his body, further explaining his chronic fatigue and pain. It was clear that his lymphatic system was struggling to cope with the waste and toxins, exacerbating his overall health issues. Understanding the gravity of his condition, Judy and I were determined to help Albert restore balance and vitality to his life.

Albert arrived for his first session feeling apprehensive about what would happen. I explained the energy bed, and he drifted off to sleep within ten minutes. He felt relaxed and confident that I would not harm him. I began working on his severely bloated and hardened intestines, which were blocking the flow of nutrient-rich plasma needed to heal the pelvic region. This blockage was also affecting his bladder function.

After just 30 minutes, his waistline had softened, and Albert was amazed by the calming and healing effects. Albert scheduled two more visits for lymphatic drainage massage, gaining more energy with each session. At the same time, his waistline continued to shrink, and his fear of cancer diminished—an issue primarily due to a lack of water, oxygen, and nutrients. By the time Albert left for his overseas trip, he was in high spirits, with his bladder and bowel functions nearly back to normal. His remarkable recovery showcased the transformative power of lymphatic therapy.

4   MIKE

What else can I do? The pain is killing me.

Mike was Jane's husband, a client of mine for several years. During our many conversations, Jane often shared details about her husband's health struggles. He had been in severe pain for over four weeks, and it was worsening. The doctors diagnosed him with pulmonary edema, a condition caused by excessive fluid in the lungs. Jane described how Mike was struggling to breathe, couldn't sleep lying down, had painful ribs, and found no relief from medication.

I told Jane to have Mike see me the next day; this situation couldn't continue. Jane chuckled and said, "You know how sceptical he is. He thinks I'm mad for coming to see you."

That afternoon, I received a phone call from Mike. Before he could start speaking, I began explaining his condition. "Mike, it's like your lungs are stuck to your rib cage with super glue. This inhibits your oxygen intake and makes you feel like you can't catch your breath."

Mike was stunned and said, "That's exactly how I feel. I can't sleep, can't lie on my side, and my job requires me to drive all over the countryside, which I can't do right now."

I asked Mike to come in the next day, and he agreed. Upon meeting him and conversing, I said, "There's nothing inherently wrong with you. The stress in your body is causing inflammation. Because you don't breathe properly, carry excess weight, and haven't exercised much in the last twenty years, your condition has worsened."

Mike was skeptical and asked, "How will this help me?"

I replied, "Trust me, it won't take long to reduce inflammation if you follow the program. And it won't cost you anything except coming to see me."

In just one session, consisting of 30 minutes in the energy bed and 30 minutes of non-surgical treatment, I worked around his rib cage on both sides and his back. Although Mike felt some initial pain during the treatment, he experienced immediate relief once the pressure was released.

Mike left the clinic able to breathe much better and with significantly less pain. He was impressed, noting that no-one else had any idea how to help him other than to suggest rest and patience for healing.

Reducing inflammation is easier than most think. If you understand its connection to tissue blockages, the body's natural energy can solve the problem.

This is your body's healing system—your lymphatic system, your built-in doctor. It works if we don't interfere with it.

That night, Mike shared with me that he was up all night, urinating frequently, and didn't sleep a wink. Initially, he thought the treatment hadn't worked. However, what was happening was his body was eliminating excess fluid to allow more oxygen to repair his cells. The next night, he slept like a baby for a full eight hours— something he hadn't done for weeks. His stress levels and pain were significantly reduced, and life seemed to be on the mend.

Mike returned for two more sessions. While it wasn't enough, it had to do, and it was a significant improvement. I also performed a non-surgical stomach lift to reduce the waste in his waistline, and in just eight days, he lost three belt holes. By following the program, he managed to get out of pain. I recommended that he come back monthly for maintenance to keep on track. As with many skeptics, the proof is in the results—this approach works.

Mike's story is a testament to the power of the lymphatic system and the importance of addressing the root causes of inflammation and pain. His journey shows that with the proper guidance and treatment, the body's natural healing mechanisms can be unlocked, leading to significant improvements in health and well-being.

Jane shared with me that Mike didn't stick to the program, which led to him relying on medication to manage the pain as it began to return. All that effort, only to stop, seems unbelievable—but that's the reality for many people. Jane has come to realize that you can't change anyone; they must want to change themselves. In her experience, this is especially true when it comes to men.

5   ISABELLA

Isabella found me through the internet, seeking relief from severe stomach and period pain. She was burdened with a significant amount of waste around her hips, a considerable load for someone of her stature. Having been teaching for eight years, Isabella was passionate about teaching children. However, the intense curriculum and the pressures of being a young, capable teacher led to immense stress as Isabella strove to excel for her students and peers.

During the Covid years, Isabella gained weight, and despite regular gym visits, the excess weight stubbornly clung to her thighs and buttocks. This exacerbated her stress and concerns about her monthly cycles, a distressingly common issue among young women. Sounds familiar.

After just one session with me, Isabella fell in love with the healing process and purchased a 10-session package. Committed to her well-being, she traveled over an hour every Saturday for ten weeks to attend our sessions. During our time together, we delved into reclaiming her ability to manage stress effectively.

The pressures of teaching, especially in the post-Covid environment, had become overwhelming for Isabella. She was dedicated to being the best teacher possible, but the added workload and the emotional toll of dealing with stressed children had pushed her beyond her limits. Watching Isabella's transformation over the ten weeks was incredibly rewarding. Gradually, she began to shed the excess weight, and her pain diminished, revealing a glimmer of hope at the end of the tunnel. Though I hadn't seen her for a few months, she eagerly planned a significant overseas trip with her father to the USA.

Isabella's journey is a testament to the power of holistic healing, commitment, and the resilience of the human spirit.

Emotional intelligence

Emotional intelligence (EI) is recognizing, understanding, managing, and utilizing emotions effectively in ourselves and others. It starts with an awareness of the frequency of emotions, which refers to the different levels or intensities of emotional experiences. Here's how it works and how it relates to healing:

1. Awareness of Emotions: Understanding the frequency of emotions means recognizing the subtle variations in how we feel. Emotions can range from low-frequency (such as sadness, fear, or anger) to high-frequency (such as joy, love, or gratitude).

Awareness of these frequencies helps us identify our emotional state and its impact on our well-being.

2. Understanding Emotions: The next step is understanding their cause and effect once we recognize our emotions. This involves exploring the reasons behind our feelings and how they influence our thoughts and behaviors. For instance, understanding that fear may be rooted in an experience can help us address it more effectively.

3. Managing Emotions: Emotion management involves regulating feelings to promote well-being and effective functioning. This doesn't mean suppressing emotions but acknowledging them and finding healthy coping methods. Techniques such as mindfulness, deep breathing, and positive self-talk can help shift emotions from a low to a high frequency.

4. Using Emotions: High-frequency emotions like love and gratitude have a powerful healing effect on the body and mind. Individuals can enhance their overall health and resilience by intentionally cultivating these emotions. This process involves focusing on positive experiences, practicing gratitude, and engaging in activities that bring joy and fulfillment.

How I can help shift individuals into a high frequency of healing

Despite it being challenging to explain, here's how I support individuals in shifting to a high frequency of healing:

- Intuitive Guidance: After Julie passed from cancer at 52, my intuitive abilities became more pronounced. While I've always had this intuition, I learned to trust and express it over time. This intuition allows me to sense what individuals need to heal, even if they aren't consciously aware of it.

- Creating a Healing Environment: I help individuals create an environment that promotes high-frequency emotions. This might involve encouraging practices that foster joy, gratitude, and love, such as meditation, visualization, or connecting with nature.

- Emotional Support: Providing emotional support is crucial. Being present, empathetic, and understanding, I help individuals feel seen and heard, which can naturally elevate their emotional frequency.

- Education and Empowerment: Educating individuals about emotional intelligence and the power of high-frequency emotions empowers them to take charge of their healing journey. Knowledge about how emotions affect health can inspire positive changes in their lives.

- Trusting the Process: Even though I can't see spirits, ghosts, or angelic lights that others might experience, my intuition guides me to support others effectively. I trust this process and encourage others to trust their inner wisdom and healing potential.

- By integrating these elements, I facilitate individuals in transitioning into a higher frequency of healing, often without their conscious awareness. This natural, intuitive approach can lead to profound and lasting transformations in their health and well-being.

- I have learned to communicate with people's innate intelligence and reprogram it to enhance wellness and regenerate cells. This remarkable process is something you can achieve, too.

6 DEB

Deb walked into my clinic in Blackburn when I was very new at practicing Applied Lymphology.

Deb was a woman in her late forties, living with significant weight challenges and showing signs of premature aging.

Deb had lap band surgery many years before and had gone through breast cancer. She had come to me to reduce her swollen legs and find an answer for her fluid retention. They were enormous, and she put in her best effort to shed some weight and reduce her waistline.

Deb introduced herself, and I found out about her emotional condition, which was heartbreaking. Deb had been a single mum most of her life, dealing with a very aggressive sister and mother and doing her best to raise two children. I didn't know where to start. I was new at this game of lymphology.

All Deb wanted was the pain to leave her legs and to be able to walk with some comfort again. Working my magic, I started lymphatic drainage massage for 30 minutes on each leg. After the session, Deb was pleasantly surprised; the pain had eased, and she booked another session.

Five years later, I still see Deb once a fortnight. Deb has lost a considerable amount of weight and is feeling energized. Although a more considerable lady, Deb now walks with ease. Her pain is minimal, and the swelling in her legs has reduced dramatically. She doesn't have a great eating plan, but she will remain disease-free because she is happy. Deb went through breast cancer treatment 10 years ago and a lap band surgery 20 years ago. She was always a big kid at school.

Her father and mother separated when she was a young child, and she was bullied for her heaviness at school, so life, in the beginning, was challenging, to begin with. The best part of being a Lymphologist is hearing these fantastic stories of people's transformations.

7   PETE

Pete, a dear friend, has been in my life for over a decade. Over the years, I watched as his eating habits deteriorated. Despite never gaining much weight, his midsection sometimes became unusually rounded and rock-hard. Pete accepted this as a normal part of aging, like many over fifty. However, this hardened belly was a red flag. The middle of our bodies is crucial; if compacted with waste and calcified, it compromises our filtering organs that work alongside the lymphatic system. This waste harbors harmful microorganisms that severely impact our life force and chi energy.

As a dedicated builder, Pete worked tirelessly—on the tools during the day and in the office late into the night. His routine included frequent snacking and evening drinks, which led to significant inflammation in his body. His snacks, often sugary foods, exacerbated the problem. Without proper education on how the body can become unwell, these habits went unnoticed until it was too late. Pete found himself frequently visiting his local GP for medication to manage his symptoms—a quick fix rather than a solution.

Though his doctor advised him to improve his diet and cut down on alcohol to lower his blood sugar levels, there was a critical oversight: the impact of stress. Cortisol, known as the "stress hormone", is produced by the adrenal glands and plays a vital role in the body's response to stress. When stress levels remain high, cortisol wreaks havoc on the body, affecting everything from metabolism to immune function.

For Pete, the real killer was the chronic stress that went unaddressed. Despite the temporary relief from medication, his underlying stress continued to take a toll on his health. His story is a powerful reminder that true wellness requires more than just treating symptoms—it demands a holistic approach that addresses the root causes of our ailments.

The role of cortisol

1. Stress Response:
   - Fight-or-Flight: When you experience stress, your body triggers the "fight-or-flight" response, a survival mechanism that prepares you to confront or flee a threat. This response involves the release of cortisol.
   - Energy Mobilization: Cortisol increases glucose (sugar) in the bloodstream by promoting gluconeogenesis, producing glucose from non-carbohydrate sources. This ensures that you have enough energy to respond to the stressor.
2. Metabolic Effects:
   - Blood Sugar Regulation: Cortisol helps regulate blood sugar levels by ensuring that your body has enough glucose available during times of stress. It counteracts insulin to prevent cells from taking too much glucose too quickly, keeping more glucose in the blood.
   - Fat and Protein Metabolism: It also plays a role in the metabolism of fats and proteins, breaking them down for energy sources.

Cortisol and disease

1. Chronic Stress and Cortisol:
   - Prolonged Elevation: While short-term cortisol release is essential for survival, chronic stress leads to prolonged elevation of cortisol levels. This can have several detrimental effects on the body.
   - Immune Suppression: High cortisol levels suppress the immune system, making the body more susceptible to infections and diseases.
   - Inflammation: Cortisol initially has anti-inflammatory effects, but chronic exposure can lead to increased inflammation, which can contribute to various chronic diseases.

2. Impact on Blood Sugar and Insulin:
   - Insulin Resistance: Persistently high cortisol levels can lead to insulin resistance, in which the body's cells become less responsive to insulin. This increases the risk of developing type 2 diabetes.
   - Fat Storage: Cortisol promotes fat storage, particularly in the abdominal area, linked to metabolic syndrome and cardiovascular diseases.

3. Other Health Issues:
   - Digestive Problems: Chronic stress and high cortisol can affect digestion, leading to issues like irritable bowel syndrome (IBS).
   - Mental Health: High cortisol levels are associated with mood disorders, such as anxiety and depression.
   - Cardiovascular Health: Elevated cortisol can increase blood pressure and contribute to cardiovascular diseases.

Pete's journey

As you can read, this is not a good place to be. If this becomes a pattern or program, it leads to illness and disease. Pete was heading down this road very quickly. Lucky for him, he knew me and had been a great businessman for 30 years. But Pete didn't listen to me thoroughly and started taking medication for his discomfort.

Pete knew what to do: exercise, drink structured water, relax, and eat nourishing food. But these were too hard to manage on the run and between emails for his bustling business, which he ran alone.

Then, one day, the pain in his foot became unbearable. The acid in his body had finally caught up with him, and it felt like a stabbing pain that wouldn't go away. Pete waited a week or two before going to the doctor, and sure enough, it was gout—the worst thing in the world.

After the pain subsided, Pete noticed a red rash on his side. Concerned, he returned to the doctor, seeking answers. The diagnosis was unexpected: the gout medication he had been prescribed had triggered a case of shingles. This revelation shocked Pete, as shingles are a side effect of the drug. The news was surprising and alarming, as shingles can lead to severe complications, including potential blindness. Pete now faced a new, daunting challenge with serious risks and uncertainties.

As a lymphologist, I knew the problem was caused by the crystallization of stored waste, which impaired blood flow and oxygenation in his tissues.

At ten o'clock at night, we drove down to the GP to get the diagnosis of gout. Medication was the first point of call—anything to get rid of this excruciating pain. I didn't say anything as it would have been brushed aside. Pete had to learn the best way to heal and go through what he was experiencing. After a few days, the pain subsided, but the side effects came on thick and fast: feeling tired, brain fog, and other little things Pete couldn't put his finger on. Pete went off alcohol for a while and gave up bread and sugary foods, and his life of pain became less intense. Life continued once again.

Six months later, back to old habits, I was working at the clinic when I received a phone call. "Michelle, can you fit me in, even for 30 minutes? The pain is so unbearable. My foot is so sore I can't even walk."

This time, Pete didn't go back to the doctor. He called me first. I said, "Sure, come down to the clinic straight away. I will fit you in."

His foot was numb and cold—a sure sign that oxygen was not entering the foot 100%, and there were blockages around the small bones of his ankle and foot. I worked on the area for 30 minutes, breaking down the calcification. Once the waste was broken up using a non-surgical technique, which I learned from Darrell Wolfe, the pain completely disappeared in 30 minutes. Pete was also lying on the E-Power Belt, a machine that boosts the body's frequency and creates more significant amounts of electricity.

From that day on, Pete realized the importance of maintaining his health properly and never looked back. He left my clinic with the clapper, a simple plastic device designed to create vibrations when struck against the body, breaking up stagnation and promoting healing.

That night, determined to relieve his chronic pain, Pete diligently used the clapper on his foot for hours. "My goodness, it hurts," he muttered, but he was astounded to see increased blood flow and feel warmth and sensation returning to his foot. The following day, he woke up pain-free, astonished that his efforts had effectively reversed his discomfort.

Although Pete has yet to master self-healing, he has come remarkably close. Although I haven't seen Pete in my clinic since that day, our paths still cross at our friendship group gatherings. I'm thrilled to report that he no longer suffers from gout pain. Hooray for Pete's incredible journey to better health!

8   GIOVANNA

I first met Giovanna in January 2024. At 80, she was a graceful and beautiful woman despite her challenges. Her friend had heard of my work as a lymphologist and, though unsure of its intricacies, believed it might help Giovanna.

Giovanna had been living with dementia and severe swelling in her right arm for over 15 years, a consequence of breast cancer surgery that resulted in the removal of her right breast. Dementia, a term encompassing over 100 different diseases, had compounded her difficulties, but her family's immediate concern was the painful swelling in her arm.

The swelling had become so severe that Giovanna couldn't fasten her bra, dress herself, or use her right arm as she wished. Her family was distraught, especially as her doctors had no answers. Desperate, they found me.

When I first met Giovanna, she was in significant pain and discomfort. The surgery from years ago had led to calcification, tightening the connective tissues. Moving her arm was like trying to stretch a dried-out rubber band.

After just one session, Giovanna felt a noticeable improvement in her overall wellness and health. To me, her condition didn't seem like a brain dysfunction but rather a lonely heart. She had lost her husband of 60 years 15 years ago, and although she lived with her grown-up son, it wasn't the same as having her husband by her side.

Giovanna's caregiver drove her to see me once a week for an hour of lymphatic drainage. During our sessions, we spoke about her childhood in Italy and her family, all of whom had passed away, leaving her the last one remaining. Giovanna looked forward to our sessions, and after just a few weeks, the swelling in her right arm had significantly reduced, and she could move it again.

In addition to lymphatic drainage, I performed non-surgical techniques to release the scar tissue under her right armpit and around her scars. Giovanna also used our energy bed, which boosted her vitamin D levels, strengthened her bones, and promoted overall health.

Giovanna had been coming to see me for about eight months when my office received a call from her daughter. Giovanna had fallen and was rushed to the hospital to check for broken bones. To the doctors' amazement, she had no broken bones, only minor bruising. Giovanna returned two weeks later to her regular lymphatic drainage and energy bed sessions.

Her case manager, who hadn't seen Giovanna since she started her sessions with Lymphology Australia, was shocked at the improvement. Her right arm looked fantastic, and the clarity of her mind showed noticeable improvement.

We had been helping Giovanna in ways we hadn't fully realized, improving her mental and physical health. Unfortunately, her carer's package funds eventually ran out, and she had to stop seeing me. However, we managed to significantly reduce her pain and improve her mobility, giving her a better quality of life.

Lymphology and healing yourself

What makes the body tick? What causes our pain? Imagine a world where we could heal from any ailment within our tissues. Picture a society where self-healing is the norm—no doctors, no medications, no inflammation. Instead, we live in harmony, driven by friendship, unconditional love, and genuine care for one another. A world free from stress and suffering, where the human spirit thrives. But as with everything in life, there are two sides to every story, and this is ours...

Teaching lymphology, which is the study of the lymphatic system, can be organized around three main topics.

1. **Anatomy and Physiology of the Lymphatic System**
   - **Structure and Components**:
     - Lymphatic vessels
     - Lymph nodes
     - Lymphoid organs (spleen, thymus, tonsils)
     - Lymph fluid
   - **Functions:**
     - Fluid balance
     - Immune system support: Absorption of fats and fat-soluble vitamins
2. **Lymphatic Diseases**
   - **Lymphedema:**
     - Primary (genetic) and secondary (caused by injury or surgery)

- ○ Symptoms and stages
- ○ Diagnosis and management
- **Lymphadenopathy**:
  - ○ Causes (infections, cancers, autoimmune diseases)
  - ○ Symptoms and treatments
- **Lymphatic Filariasis**:
  - ○ Parasitic infection
  - ○ Epidemiology, prevention, and treatment

3. **Lymphatic Health and Therapies**
   - **Lymphatic Drainage Techniques**:
     - ○ Manual lymphatic drainage (MLD)
     - ○ Compression therapy
     - ○ Exercise and movement
   - **Lifestyle and Dietary Considerations**:
     - ○ Diet and nutrition for lymphatic health
     - ○ Hydration
     - ○ Avoiding toxins and maintaining a healthy lifestyle
   - **Emerging Therapies and Research**:
     - ○ Advances in medical treatments
     - ○ Research in lymphatic function and disorders

These topics provide a comprehensive framework for teaching lymphology, encompassing the fundamental aspects of the lymphatic system, its associated disorders, and how to maintain and improve lymphatic health.

The art of healing is a way of life. Why do some people heal and others don't? Why do some people take longer to heal than others? This is the million-dollar question in every practice worldwide, from Western to Eastern medicine.

K +
Na +

Glucose
+   = A.T.P
Oxygen

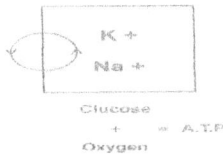

Oxygen = Pumps = Electricity = Power

DRY STATE

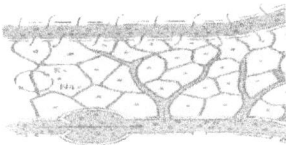

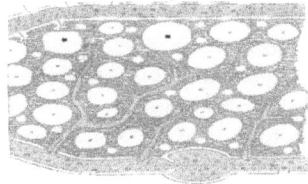

MENTAL
Love, Bless
Do Good
Desire to Give
All to Bless Others

NUTRITIONAL

More
Fruits
Vegetables
Grains
Fish
(No Thirst—
Energy High)

PHYSICAL

Breathe Deeply
and
Exercise Properly
(Lymphasize)
(Energy High)

MENTAL
Shock, Stress, Anger
Fear, Loss of Temper,
Holding Grudges
Resentment, Greed

NUTRITIONAL

Tea, Coffee, Liquor,
Tobacco, Soft Drinks
Drugs, Salt, Sugar, Fat
High Cholesterol Foods
Too Much Meat
(Thirst and
Loss of Energy)

PHYSICAL

Shallow Breathing
and
Improper Exercise
(Loss of Energy)

Printed with permission Professor Karl West

The art of Lymphology was first introduced by C Samuel West, the Golden Seven Plus One, who conquered disease with eight keys to health, beauty, and peace. Peace is the number one rule in his teaching and mine. Without peace, we have no friendship. Without friendship, how can we love the community? How can we respect, honor, and love each other unconditionally? Imagine the entire world as one body: a community of thousands of cells, all sharing the same space, oxygen, food nutrition, micro-organisms, and general flora and fauna that are part of the human body. Imagine the disharmony if each of those cells fought each other. We wouldn't survive one day!

9 LUKE

The mysterious return of Luke – the unexpected call

In July 2024, a familiar yet unexpected name re-entered my life—Luke. I had never met him before, but a strange and fascinating event occurred in 2016. Sean and I then shared a space in Blackburn, Melbourne, offering lymphatic drainage and energy wellness therapies. Luke was one of Sean's clients, a man who had left an indelible impression on Sean.

My office manager, Judy, answered the phone that day. The man on the other end had a calm, gentle voice. "I'd like to book a session for the SOQI energy bed," he said. "I did a few sessions with Sean before Covid." Judy was puzzled, unsure of who this mysterious caller was. She relayed the conversation to me, and a flicker of recognition sparked in my mind. Could it be the same Luke who had been Sean's client all those years ago?

Judy scheduled the appointment, but I couldn't shake the feeling that this was more than a simple session booking. Luke had explicitly requested the energy bed and wanted a session for his uncle. The details were intriguing, and I was eager to see where this encounter would lead.

Luke walked in accompanied by his uncle. They introduced themselves, and immediately, I was struck by the aura of familiarity surrounding Luke. As we exchanged pleasantries, Luke's eyes seemed to hold secrets from the past, secrets I was about to uncover.

He began to recount his experiences from Blackburn. "I remember you wrote out an assessment for me on a handheld frequency device," he said. "Everything you noted about my life was astonishingly accurate. You had never met me before, yet you knew so much about me. How did you do it?"

I listened intently, my curiosity piqued. The device he mentioned was something we had used extensively before the pandemic, but we had since discontinued its use. Memories of those days flooded back, and with them, a sense of mystery. How could I have known so much about Luke without ever meeting him?

As Luke and his uncle settled into their sessions, I couldn't help but reflect on our strange connection. The SOQI energy bed hummed softly, enveloping the room in a gentle, healing energy. I watched as Luke closed his eyes, serenity washing over his face.

After the session, Luke approached me once more.

"You have a gift," he said, his voice filled with awe. "The things you wrote about my life—they were all true. It's as if you had a window into my soul."

I smiled, touched by his words but also deeply curious. "Sometimes, intuition and energy guide us in ways we can't fully explain," I replied, "but there's more to this story, isn't there? Something brought you back here after all these years."

Luke nodded, his expression turning serious. "There is something," he admitted. "I've been searching for answers, trying to understand the connection we share. There's a mystery here, one that involves more than just the energy sessions."

As Luke and his uncle left after their one session, a sense of peace settled over me. Luke's return was not just a reunion; it was a reminder of the incredible potential within us all to uncover the mysteries of our own lives and to heal in ways we never imagined possible. And so, our journey continued, guided by intuition, bound by the energy that connected us, and illuminated by the light of understanding, and reminding me that I was that gift.

10 DARREN

When Darren walked into my life again, it was as if time had bent back on itself. I hadn't seen him since I was 18, when he had been my first real love. When we met, I was a humble, shy 16-year-old, enchanted by his red car and the thrill of our young romance. I had no idea what I was getting into.

Seeing him book an appointment at my clinic after over 37 years was shocking. Although he had changed, the memories rushed back. Unsure whether to shake his hand or embrace him, I asked, "What brought you here?"

Darren hesitated. "I almost didn't come. But your story on social media... I hoped you could help me put my body back together."

"Is that all?" I replied, laughing. "Of course, I can help." We shared a genuine, hearty laugh.

Darren was severely overweight, his posture was misaligned, and he was far from the young man I once knew. As he began to recount his life, my heart ached. Our two-year relationship had been magical until he suddenly ended it, telling me I deserved someone better. I was heartbroken and left in total disbelief.

At 57, Darren's heart was still shattered. He revealed that his father had beaten and abused him from a young age. He had never told me this during our time together. I remembered his parents being a bit strange, but I thought nothing of it as a young girl.

Over the next six months, Darren visited weekly for lymphatic drainage massages. I taught him the importance of rebounding and core strength, slowly uncovering and reversing his pain. His story, locked away for too long, had been destroying his body and soul.

Not long after our breakup, Darren had a significant car accident that left him in constant pain, and believing his body was unlovable. He had never had another girlfriend, children, or a fulfilling life. He had fallen into a life of isolation and loneliness.

As Darren shared his story, I realized the profound impact of our reconnection. Our laughter, tears, and the healing process we embarked on together brought a sense of closure and a new beginning. Darren's journey back to health and self-love was a testament to the power of resilience and the human spirit.

Then Covid hit hard, and Darren's worries escalated. He decided to stop visiting the clinic, fearing for his safety. Over the last two years, Darren suffered two strokes and various other health issues, struggling to regain his footing in life. Despite receiving two Covid-19 vaccines, he remained isolated, terrified of falling gravely ill. During the pandemic, I lost touch with Darren; it was a harrowing time for many.

In 2023, out of the blue, his sister called. She revealed that Darren had suffered another stroke and was now in the ICU ward in Melbourne. His prognosis was uncertain.

11   KIM

The lost voice

Kim entered my clinic searching for answers to her lost voice and confidence. Kim was a beautiful young woman of 50, having played many roles across the TV screens in our lounge rooms. Kim was searching to fill a gap in her life; something profound was missing. With no children and a childhood spent in the theatre with her mother as the center stage, Kim's life had been a whirlwind of travel and constant change. Kim loved watching her mother perform, inspiring her to pursue acting. However, her life as a young girl lacked stability. The acting bug ran in the family, even extending to her grandmother.

Kim would be complex, as her belief system was intertwined with low self-esteem. Approaching age 50, she felt overshadowed by younger actors pursuing their careers and leaving their marks on the screen. Although Kim was still offered significant roles, she seemed to lack the confidence she once had.

Her body was super tight with tension, and the inflammation was sky-high. Kim didn't realize this was a side effect of her emotional state. She oscillated between feeling fabulous and not so good. Once I gained her trust, Kim opened up about her world of low self-esteem and emptiness. It was ironic that someone who had been seen on the screen for most of her life felt so inadequate.

Kim loved the SOQI bed and the information about the lymphatic drainage session. She was intrigued by how it would help eliminate waste in her body. Like many others, Kim didn't realize that garbage carries all our emotions stored in our cells. I assured her she would feel lighter and more at peace with past traumas.

As I worked on her, I started sharing insights about what she was holding onto. Kim was astonished and asked how I knew. I just smiled and continued my role, helping her see the damage she was doing to herself by holding onto a belief that she wasn't good enough.

Kim attended several sessions and was excited to return each time, saying that the old Kim was returning. It was fantastic, but something was happening, and Kim would slip back into her old habits, though not as far as before. I focused on her shoulders, heart release, and the large intestine area, which was full of emotional baggage. Every time Kim left after a session, she was full of life and keen to return to her acting career and find her voice again. It was frustrating, as her subconscious habits wouldn't let her fully move forward.

Breaking the chains

The process was slow but steady. Kim's sessions became a journey of self-discovery and healing. We delved deeper into her childhood, her experiences on the road, and the pressures of living up to her family's legacy. Each session was a step towards breaking the chains of her past and building a new foundation of self-worth.

We incorporated meditation and mindfulness exercises to reconnect Kim with her inner self. I encouraged her to journal her thoughts and feelings, which helped her identify patterns and triggers. This helped Kim see the connection between her emotions and her physical state.

Kim's progress was evident. Her posture improved, the tension in her body lessened, and she started radiating a newfound confidence. Kim began taking on roles that challenged her and brought back the passion she once felt for acting.

However, setbacks were inevitable. There were days when the old doubts resurfaced, and Kim felt herself slipping back. During these times, we focused on reinforcing her progress and reminding her of the strength she had within. It was a continuous battle that Kim was now equipped to resolve.

The transformation

Kim's transformation was not just physical, but emotional, and spiritual. She learned to forgive herself for past mistakes and to let go of the unrealistic expectations she had placed on herself. She embraced her journey, acknowledging that healing was not linear but filled with ups and downs.

The culmination of Kim's journey was a significant role she landed in a new series. This role was different; it resonated with her newfound sense of self. It wasn't just about acting, but expressing her truth and healing journey. The role allowed her to connect with her audience deeper, sharing her vulnerability and strength.

Kim's story inspired many. She began speaking about her experiences, helping others who felt lost and inadequate. Once silenced by doubt, her voice became a beacon of hope and empowerment.

Ultimately, Kim discovered her voice both in acting and life, realizing that her true worth was not defined by the roles she played on screen but by the person she had become through her transformative healing journey.

A new beginning

Kim's journey is a testament to the power of healing and self-discovery. It reminds us that no matter how lost we feel, there is always a way back to our true selves. With the support of others and the courage to face our inner demons, we can overcome any obstacle and find our voice again.

This book is dedicated to all those who feel lost and those who help them find their way. May Kim's story inspire you to embark on your journey of healing and self-discovery.

12   DIANE

Di had two Covid 19 vaccines to keep her job and a roof over her head. This decision marked the beginning of a descent into hospitalization, endless doctor visits, tests upon tests, heart failure, and a bleak uncertainty about whether Di would ever return to her beloved tennis and her life at 63.

Di had always been fit, strong, and full of life, weathering life's ups and downs without complaint. But November 2021 was a day that would etch itself into her memory forever. Di didn't want another shot. She felt a deep, unshakable uncertainty about it all, but had no choice; she had to go through with it. Her gut told her this would end badly, and it did.

Two weeks after the second vaccine was injected into her body, Di collapsed on the floor. November 2021 was the day her life changed irrevocably.

Desperately trying to hold herself together, Di was rushed to the hospital only to hear the devastating words, "We don't know what's wrong with you." Two agonizing weeks in the hospital, plagued by heart issues and the sense that her world was crumbling around her, left Di feeling more isolated than ever. No-one was allowed to see her. All Di wanted was for it to be over, to escape the relentless pain and die.

They decided to inject radioactive glucose into her body and scan her heart, only to make things worse. Di felt utterly betrayed and abandoned, left alone in her ailing body with no way out. The hopelessness was overwhelming, and she struggled to find a reason to keep fighting.

Di wasn't going to die, but it felt like it. Her health was deteriorating, and the doctors had no answers. Desperation led her to seek alternatives. She embarked on a journey into integrative health, consulting a naturopath who prescribed costly natural vitamins. Di also sought relief from an acupuncturist, but the pain in her knees and back persisted despite some improvement. Di felt trapped, losing hope.

One day, while shopping, she struck up a conversation with a stranger about her pain. The stranger suggested seeing a lymphatic drainage massage therapist. Di decided to try it with dwindling finances and nothing left to lose.

In December 2023, Di's life changed forever. After just one session of lymphatic massage, her pain vanished. Astonished, She asked, "How did you do that?"

I smiled, "It's my job to educate and communicate with your innate wisdom, clearing the blockages that cause pain."

Di's curiosity was piqued. "Please explain," she requested.

I began, "We are electric beings of energy, powered by a life force that runs through the universe. This force governs everything—the earth, the rain, the sun, the wind, and the tides. We often take this for granted, but it's the essence of our existence. We are here to experience heaven on earth, but we sometimes lose sight of the peace within and around us. This disconnection causes dis-ease, creating resentment in our lives, families, workplaces, and partnerships."

This disconnection fractures us, spiraling us into emotional pain and heartache. Your innate intelligence seeks one thing: unconditional love and peace. When you embrace this, you can let go of the pain."

Di absorbed these words, realizing their profound truth. Her journey wasn't just about physical healing and reconnecting with her inner self and the universe. She began to see her pain as a signal, a guide to a deeper understanding and a more profound transformation.

This began Di's new life of healing, understanding, and embracing the universal energy that connects us all. Her story, shared with billions, became a testament to the power of integrative health and the incredible potential of the human spirit.

Di herself – a letter to Senator Hansen-Young & Senator Waters

I am writing to you both to express my disgust, anger, and extreme disappointment with your appalling and disgraceful behavior in Parliament last week. While Senator Gerard Rennick was making a speech about vaccine injuries and lifting mandates, both of you heckled him.

I am one of the many thousands of people who have been maimed and permanently injured by the Covid-19 vaccinations. My health and quality of life have been destroyed by this shot, which I had in good faith after consulting and trusting my GP and health authorities; how very wrong was I, and now for the rest of my life, along with thousands of others, will be paying the price. I had my second AZ Vax on the 30th of November last year. That afternoon, I felt unwell. Two days later, the glands in my throat swelled, and I was prescribed antibiotics; after two weeks, I still felt highly unwell, so my GP sent me to have an urgent blood test, which showed I had suspected blood clots and an infection somewhere in my body. The following day, 17th December 2021, I momentarily passed out at home and had

*heart palpitations and sweaty palms. I was taken by ambulance
to the hospital and spent the next two weeks having extensive
harrowing tests done and missed out on Christmas with my
family. I was discharged on 30th December. I had suspected
Myocarditis. Every day a nurse came to administer antibiotics
into a drip in my arm.*

*Most nights I had to sleep sitting upright in a chair due to the
severe chest pains I was experiencing when lying down.*

*Then, in late January this year, my joints became swollen
and painful. I had further blood tests, which showed I had
Rheumatoid Arthritis; I then had to take steroid medication to
combat the pain, which came with serious side effects.*

*Before the vax, I had excellent health, played tennis for over
45 years, and led an active and independent life. I am now 100%
certain that the vax caused my severe health issues and triggered
the autoimmune disease in me. I am now losing my hair because of
the medication I take for the treatment of RA. My rheumatologist
said RA can also cause alopecia.*

*I can now do very little without feeling extraordinarily
fatigued. Since I live alone, it is challenging as I no longer have the
quality of life and independence I had before I was vaccinated. You
may or may not know there is no cure for Rheumatoid Arthritis. It
is a highly debilitating disease, and it comes with extreme fatigue.
The vaccination is not safe and effective for everyone, and it should
never have been mandated. It was highly toxic and dangerous for
me, and as a result, I no longer have the quality of life and good
health I had before being vaccinated. Before being vaccinated,
I lived an active and independent life and was healthy. This is
no longer the case; my mental and physical health has suffered*

enormously. As a result, I am seeing a psychologist to help me with the mental anguish and grief that I suffer as a result of what the vax has done to me. I have also been seeing a naturopath to try and improve my health somewhat, and being an age pensioner, that can be difficult to afford. Going by your actions and your abhorrent behavior in parliament by laughing and mocking the vax injured and Senator Hansen-Young had the gall to move that the debate be shut down, it shows me your lack of respect and compassion and how insensitive you are to people like me and the thousands of others who suffered and who have been permanently maimed and injured as a result of the Covid vaccinations.

Regards Dianne P

After just a few months of lymphatic drainage massage, Di has now reclaimed her life, freed herself from all medications, and is stepping back into a vibrant and empowered life. Di followed the program.

13   ROB

The unknown watcher

Social media has always been a tool I used to build my clientele. My sister would always say to me, "You spend so much time on it," and I often found myself echoing, "You never know who is watching." Little did I know, someone was indeed watching. His name was Rob, and he was halfway across the world in the Philippines.

It was late night when Rob first reached out to me. The message came through Facebook, and as I read it, I could sense the desperation in his words. "Michelle, can you help me? I am in incredible pain, hours from the local hospital, and I really don't want to go. They don't speak English, and I don't want them to put anything into me, but the pain is unbearable."

I immediately responded, setting up a video call. When Rob appeared on my screen, his face was a mask of agony. He was sweating profusely, and every movement seemed to send a wave of pain through his body. Despite the distance, I knew I had to help him.

As we began our call, it became clear that Rob was severely dehydrated and struggling to breathe. Every time he moved, the pain would stab at him, making it difficult for him to remain calm. The first thing I needed to do was get him to breathe properly. "Rob, just take nice, slow breaths for me," I instructed. "There's nothing wrong with you that we can't fix."

Rob tried to follow my instructions, but he was scared. His breaths were shallow and rapid, and his body tensed with each air intake. I continued reassuring him calmly and steadily. "You're going to be okay, Rob. Just breathe. Nice and slow."

Gradually, he began to relax. His breathing relaxed, and tension seemed to melt away with each exhale. "That's it, Rob," I encouraged, "keep breathing just like that." As he continued to breathe more deeply, the pain started to subside, little by little.

With Rob more relaxed, we could focus on the next steps. I guided him through simple hydration techniques, instructing him to sip water slowly. He kept the water down, and his color soon improved. "You're doing great, Rob," I said. Now, let's see if we can ease that pain more."

I guided him through gentle movements and stretches to help alleviate some of the discomfort. It was a slow process, but with each small success, Rob's confidence grew. We spent a short amount of time on that call, working through each wave of pain and fear together.

By the end of our session, Rob was sitting up more comfortably, breathing steadily, and the pain had diminished significantly. "Thank you, Michelle," he said, his voice filled with gratitude. "I don't know what I would have done without you."

This experience reminded me of the incredible power of connection and the human spirit. Despite the distance and circumstances, we found a way to heal together. It was a testament to our strength and resilience and a reminder that sometimes, a little guidance and compassion can make a significant difference.

14   DAINA AND KAREN

February 2023: the arrival

Daina drove Karen to my clinic, their home just down the road. Karen was a cancer patient at the Alfred Hospital. As she entered my room, her frail frame and fearful eyes reflected the looming end she knew was approaching, though she didn't know when. Karen, only 52 years old, looked much older. She had never married, had no children, and had spent her life caring for her mother. The sisters, Daina and Karen, shared a deep, bitter rivalry, each resenting the other.

In a private conversation, Daina expressed her frustration with caring for Karen. She longed to focus on her own life and her beloved dogs. Their father lived nearby on the Peninsula, while the sisters remained in the parental home, constantly battling over their late mother's inheritance. This ongoing conflict deeply affected Karen.

I welcomed Karen into my clinic, explaining how our sessions would proceed. Karen looked at me pleadingly, saying, "Michelle, I wish for the pain to subside. I'm not looking for a miracle, just relief. I'm still under my doctors' care, receiving monthly injections, but they seem to cause more pain and exhaustion. Can you help me?"

Though this was heart-wrenching, my training as a lymphologist under Samuel West, founder of LLS, taught me to practice unconditional love without attachment and to understand that energy and spirit are eternal.

"Okay, Karen," I said, "I'll release the waste in your body to allow oxygen in and facilitate repair. However, the strong drugs you're on might interfere with our sessions." Despite my concerns, I resolved to treat her gently, mindful of her fragile state.

During our first session, I addressed Karen with the utmost care, unaware of her bone density condition. To my relief, she experienced a reduction in pain and a newfound calmness. Karen had longed for the tender love in my touch all her life. She had no-one, which reminded me of my lonely upbringing as a triplet.

Surprisingly, Karen's energy began to return, and even Daina noticed a difference. Karen, an accomplished artist and woodworker, started to show me her impressive creations. Over the next two months, Karen attended twice-weekly lymphatic drainage massage sessions. Near the end of this period, she hesitantly mentioned, "Michelle, I'm due for my medication injection next week. I feel so amazing; maybe I shouldn't get it."

I advised her to follow her intuition, as I couldn't tell her what to do. Her doctors noticed her progress and were pleased with her improvement.

However, Karen decided to have her monthly check-up and injection. After missing a session, she called me, sounding weak and exhausted. "Michelle, I had the injection and now I feel so sick and tired. I told them I was feeling better and wanted to skip it this month, but they insisted."

The final days

Karen spent the next two days in the hospital, too ill to move. When she finally returned to me, she could only manage two more sessions. Traveling had become a significant challenge, and her body was shutting down. After our last session, I never heard from Karen or Daina again.

Despite our brief time together, I felt grateful to have given Karen a glimpse of unconditional love and relief. Through our conversations and the healing touch, she experienced something magical. Although her journey ended sooner than hoped, Karen had tasted a new lease on life, if only temporarily.

Reflecting on this, I realized that the power of love and lymphology can make a profound difference, even in the face of the most heartbreaking circumstances. As I continued my work, Karen's memory remained with me, a reminder of the impact one has on another's life, however fleeting.

15   PAUL

Paul's journey was nothing short of extraordinary. Burdened by excruciating hip pain and the fear of invasive surgery, he arrived at the brink of despair. Yet, through courage, commitment, and the power of true healing, Paul's transformation became a testament to what's possible when the body and soul are given the chance to thrive.

Paul found me through an online search, driven by curiosity and desperation. He had read countless testimonials of others who had found relief through my sessions, and though he was hesitant, his chronic pain left him with few options. After years of suffering and countless visits to physiotherapists that only provided temporary relief, Paul decided to leap into faith.

When Paul arrived for his first session, his skepticism was evident. He had spent years trying different treatments, each promising to be the solution, yet none provided lasting results. His pain always returned, and the financial burden of constant therapy visits was wearing him down. I could see the exhaustion in his eyes and the weariness in his posture.

As we began, I explained to Paul that his pain stemmed from postural alignment issues and the cellular memories of past traumas that were interfering with his healing. Paul stared at me, a mix of confusion and disbelief on his face. "Are you nuts?" he asked, half-jokingly, trying to mask his doubt.

I responded with a warm smile, "Yes, perhaps," and we both laughed, breaking the tension in the room.

Paul's story unfolded as we talked. Paul had been out of an abusive marriage for five years and was raising his 12-year-old daughter alone. The responsibility of being a single parent was immense, but Paul was devoted to his daughter and determined to give her the best life possible. However, the persistent pain was eroding his spirit, making the daily challenges even more complicated to bear.

As I assessed Paul, I immediately noticed the misalignment in his back. The calcification at the junction of his coccyx bone and the thoracic and sacral vertebral segments was restricting the flow of spinal fluid, contributing to his physical and emotional distress. Before he even spoke, I knew what needed to be addressed.

I placed Paul in the SOQI bed for thirty minutes, allowing him to relax deeply. The bed's soothing warmth and gentle vibrations eased his tension. When he emerged, I could see a hint of relief on his face, but the real work was just beginning.

We faced his deepest fear together: the feeling of not being good enough. By addressing this emotional barrier, we set the stage for proper healing. Paul lay on his back as I performed a non-surgical therapy to release the calcification in his lower spine. This technique, taught by Darrel Wolfe and his son Sage Wolfe from the USA, has transformed many lives. The precise process required a deep understanding of the body's intricate systems.

As I worked on Paul, I could feel the tension in his body gradually release. The knots of pain and emotional trauma began to unwind. After an hour of lymphatic drainage massage and non-surgical intervention, Paul stood up, pain-free for the first time in years.

He was incredulous. After just one session, years of suffering had finally ended. His eyes welled up with tears of relief and gratitude. "I can't believe it," he kept repeating, shaking his head in disbelief.

Paul returned for several more sessions, showing remarkable posture improvement and pain reduction each time. His monthly visits became a time to catch up and address any lingering emotional issues. As his body healed, so did his mind, shedding layers of emotional trauma. Paul shared stories of his daughter's achievements, his renewed energy to engage in life, and the joy of being pain-free.

Paul's pain was gone in just four sessions, and he was ready to embrace life again. His transformation was not just physical but emotional and mental as well. The once-doubtful man had become a testament to the power of holistic healing and the loss of many belt sizes around his waist. Paul's journey was a confirmation of the power of addressing physical and emotional pain. His transformation was remarkable, and he became a living example of what true healing can achieve. With his newfound strength and resilience, Paul was not only able to be the father his daughter needed but also a source of inspiration to those around him. His story spread, encouraging others to seek the healing they desperately needed. Through Paul, I saw the ripple effect of true healing. One person's journey to wellness had the power to inspire and uplift countless others. It reminded me why I had dedicated my life to this work. Every session, every story, every transformation was a step toward a world where people could live free from pain and full of hope.

16   WENDY

Eight months ago, Wendy entered my clinic with her carer. She was engulfed in relentless pain. Wendy, an 81-year-old woman with an indomitable spirit and formidable mind, had endured a decade of trials. Ten years prior, she lost her husband of 55 years, an event that shattered her world. Soon after, she faced a diagnosis of breast cancer. Her doctors removed her left breast and subjected her to six grueling months of chemotherapy and radiation. Despite the sickness and suffering, Wendy was resolute in her fight against cancer, determined to overcome the agony that plagued her body.

The grief from losing her husband was a torment she could scarcely bear. Wendy recounted how his absence felt like a sudden, irrevocable void—one moment, he was there; the next, he was gone. Even a decade later, boxes from their shared life remained untouched, remnants of a past filled with love. Wendy's life brimmed with the joy of her grandchildren, and she helped around the house whenever she could, contributing to her family's well-being.

Under the care of her local doctor, Wendy managed her medication and the aftermath of her cancer diagnosis. However, her doctor could offer little relief from the persistent pain, especially the excruciating discomfort in her middle back and under her armpit, where her breast had been removed. Embracing an integrative approach to healthcare, her doctor recommended lymphatic drainage therapy. A search on Google led Wendy to my clinic, buoyed by my positive reviews.

Wendy arrived in debilitating pain, with limited movement in her left arm due to years of scar tissue accumulation from her surgery. The tissue had hardened, becoming tight and unbearably painful. Desperate to avoid heavy painkillers, Wendy sought an alternative path to relief.

We discussed her condition, and I offered not a miracle but an understanding of her body's plight and a plan to alleviate her pain. From a lymphologist's perspective, the key was reducing scar tissue and restoring blood flow to facilitate cellular repair. Wendy's upper back muscles were so tight they caused a pronounced curvature in her thoracic spine, leading to constricted chest muscles.

In our first session, Wendy experienced remarkable relief. The pain diminished, and she felt a glimmer of hope. She sent me a heartfelt message, expressing her gratitude for the respite from pain. While I knew the pain would likely return due to the severity of her scar tissue, we remained hopeful that we could manage it to improve her quality of life.

Wendy attended four one-hour sessions weekly. Gradually, the pain lessened, a triumph for both Wendy and me. A few months later, during a routine check-up, Wendy's doctor noted her excellent blood work, declaring her free of cancer and off medication. Wendy was elated, her pain significantly reduced, and her health improved.

Depending on her stress levels, Wendy's pain fluctuated but never reverted to the unbearable stabbing she once endured. Now, she visits every two to three weeks, finding solace in the therapeutic massages and our conversations, which nurture her mental and physical well-being.

17   FRAN

The journey begins

Fran walked into my clinic with a palpable determination. Her primary goal was to shed the stubborn weight that had clung to her body over the years. More than just the excess pounds, Fran struggled with fluid retention, commonly known as "cankles" – swelling around the ankles and calf muscles. This fluid buildup was a clear sign of an overburdened lymphatic system.

The calf, often called the "second brain," is crucial in activating the lymphatic system. The journey starts at the calf muscle, which pumps a vacuum-like force throughout the body. The muscle pushes waste through lymph nodes and processes it through the bladder and bowel. The rest is purified into water and re-enters the heart to start the cycle anew.

Fran, in her early sixties, was seeing multiple therapists to address her fluid retention and body pain. She knew she was carrying too much weight for her frame, but like many of us, the extra pounds had crept up gradually until everyday tasks became a struggle. Her clothes were tight, and even fastening a bra became challenging.

During our initial sessions, Fran talked about her life, revealing that stress was a significant factor in her inflammation and fluid retention. In just one session, Fran noticed a difference in her ankles. The gentle lymphatic massage was encouraging her body to heal. Intrigued by the results, Fran committed to visiting me every fortnight and rejoined her local gym, Curves.

As we continued our sessions, Fran mentioned that she was having trouble sleeping and had been diagnosed with sleep apnea. There are two main types of sleep apnoea:

- Obstructive Sleep Apnoea (OSA): Where airway obstruction leads to pauses in breathing.
- Central Sleep Apnoea (CSA): Where the brain fails to send proper signals to muscles controlling breathing.

This diagnosis was a significant concern for Fran, so she eventually began using a Continuous Positive Airway Pressure (CPAP) machine. This device provides a steady stream of air through a mask, keeping the airways open during sleep. While it was an aid, not a cure, Fran found that she slept better and snored less.

Through our conversations and sessions, we hypothesized that her nose's scar tissue contributed to her sleep apnoea. I began non-surgical treatments around her nose and face, and soon, the monitor on her CPAP machine showed that Fran needed less supplemental oxygen. She also started participating in weekly park runs, noticing an improvement in her breathing and lung capacity.

Over time, Fran reduced her visits to once a month. She is still using her CPAP machine but is feeling great overall. The confidence the machine gave her at night translated into more energy and enjoyment during the day.

Embracing the new life

As a Lymphologist, I always aim to find the best solution for everyone. I don't enforce my methods; I discover what works best for each person. Fran found her path to wellness through lymphatic therapy, physical activity, and the CPAP machine.

By the end of our journey together, Fran had lost weight, reduced her stress levels, and improved her sleep quality. Although she still used the CPAP machine, her life had transformed significantly. Fran embraced her newfound energy and joy, making the most of her days with a renewed zest for life.

Fran's happy ending was not just in losing weight or improving her sleep but in reclaiming her life. Her determination and commitment paid off, allowing her to live a more vibrant life. Seeing Fran's transformation was a testament to the power of personalized care and the incredible resilience of the human body. Fran's story reminds us that with the proper support and determination, anyone can overcome their health challenges and find their path to well-being.

18   DAVID

David's journey: a story of healing and hope

David was born a healthy baby, with all his bodily functions normal. However, after his early vaccinations, his mother began noticing changes in his development. Managing the household was already challenging with two older brothers, and David's increasingly erratic behavior added to the strain. His mother, Mrs. R, found herself exhausted, balancing the demands of her older sons with the full-time care David required.

Mrs. R was in a loving marriage, and her husband, who worked tirelessly to support the family, saw David's condition as manageable. But she knew otherwise. David's behavior grew more aggressive, especially at school, and the future seemed daunting and uncertain for both David and his mother.

Despite his challenges, David had a heart of gold. When I met him, he seemed unsure, and his communication was slow, almost as if no-one was home. However, I saw a different side of David as I connected with his innate spirit.

I need to explain this—it's a gift from the universe, and I hope to share it without sounding boastful. From a very young age, I had an uncanny ability to communicate with people, whether young, old, mentally impaired, or just different. My upbringing taught me to love everyone equally. It may sound unbelievable, but I had a unique ability to read the spirits of others. Initially, I thought I was the crazy one, but I realized that people's judgments are shaped by their perspectives and upbringing. Despite my tough childhood, I chose love over hate. I might not have shown it as a young girl, but my path was set, guided by my visions and dreams.

Some might call it a gift from God, though I am not religious. I could feel the energy around a person's body—an electric pulse of life that was truly magical. When helping people with their issues, I remained utterly present, allowing peace to envelop them. This is where the magic happened: in the peace and calm, healing and regeneration of cells took place. The body became young again, but first, I needed to lift the waste out of the cellular memory by assisting the lymphatic system. This blockage was not in the symptoms visible on the physical body but deep within. I can't fully explain it—it's an action I don't control but simply allow. And it works.

The struggle for recognition

David was a competent young man, his mind a maze of brilliance and potential, yet he was deeply impressionable, shaped by other school kids' behaviors and judgments. David's life was a landscape of loneliness and fear in the outside world. Every day was a battle against the unknown, a struggle to fit into a world that seemed to reject him at every turn. The constant barrage of social pressures and the often harsh realities of life left him feeling isolated and misunderstood.

Inside, however, David's world was entirely different. It was a sanctuary of peace and beauty where he felt safe and loved. This internal refuge was his escape, a mental cocoon where he could be himself without fear of judgment or ridicule. But this sanctuary was also a prison that isolated him from the rest of the world. David stayed in this self-imposed exile, allowing no-one in until he met me.

David's mother was desperate for him to see us once a week. She recognized our services' profound impact on her son and saw the potential for growth and healing, the chance for David to bridge the gap between his internal and external worlds. However, there was a significant obstacle in our way. Under government regulations, our services were not recognized as legitimate health services. This lack of recognition meant families like David's couldn't access funding to support these critical interventions.

The government readily funded social workers, GPs, and physiotherapists. These professionals had their value, but what we offered was unique. It was a service rooted in real-life experiences, a gift to the community that couldn't be easily quantified or categorized. Convincing the government of our value was a Herculean task fraught with frustration and bureaucratic red tape.

Despite the apparent benefits, our work remains unrecognized and unsupported by the powers. It is a constant struggle to get those in positions of authority to understand our services' truly transformative impact. We knew that if given the chance, we could change lives, helping people like David break free from their mental prisons, so they could engage with the world meaningfully.

However, a significant barrier was a lack of formal training from a recognized institution. Our expertise came from real-life experiences, countless hours working with individuals and families, and witnessing firsthand the profound changes that could occur with the proper support and intervention. While this practical knowledge was invaluable, it was not enough to meet the stringent criteria set by the government.

Our journey was one of persistent advocacy, constantly pushing against the boundaries of a system that failed to see the whole picture. It was about fighting for recognition, not for our sake but for the countless individuals who could benefit from our services. It was about giving people a choice, the opportunity to access a deeply personal and uniquely effective type of care.

David's story was just one of many, a testament to the potential locked within so many individuals who simply needed the right key to unlock their full potential. It was a story of hope and frustration, of the relentless pursuit of a dream where everyone could access the support they needed, regardless of bureaucratic hurdles.

Ultimately, it was about making things right and ensuring everyone could choose to receive services like ours. It was a battle worth fighting, a cause worth every ounce of effort because the lives we touched were worth it. And so, we continued to push forward, driven by the belief that one day, our value would be recognized, and the doors of opportunity would be opened wide for all who needed them.

19   ANDREA

A chance encounter in Coffs Harbour

The world was still grappling with the aftershocks of the pandemic when I decided to venture to Coffs Harbour, New South Wales. It was a bold decision, driven by my quest to deepen my understanding of life coaching and earn a Non-Surgical Certification under Darrell Wolfe. The course promised a transformative experience, and as I arrived, I found myself amongst twenty-seven other like-minded individuals from across the globe, all united by a common purpose: to make a difference in people's lives through this unique therapy.

The curriculum was intense, spanning over four weeks of rigorous learning. We delved deep into the intricacies of tissue calcification and the pervasive impact of inflammation on the body's healing processes.

This knowledge seamlessly complemented my lymphatic drainage massage and Lymphology expertise, which I had been practicing at my clinic with remarkable success.

During this course, I met Andrea, a fellow student from Melbourne, Victoria. At first, I found her a bit peculiar and struggled to connect with her. She seemed distant, and her demeanor was hard to read. Andrea was a mother of two teenage boys, starting her family later in life. Initially, I assumed Andrea was much older than her biological age, a misconception that puzzled me until I learned her story halfway through the course.

Andrea had been diagnosed with a severe form of cancer, a disease that doctors had deemed incurable. Their prognosis was grim, suggesting only a managed approach to prolong her life. Rejecting the conventional Western medication route, Andrea sought a natural way to combat her illness. Her diagnosis in June 2021 came right in the middle of the relentless Covid-19 lockdowns in Melbourne, a city that experienced some of the harshest restrictions globally. This compounded her challenges, creating a daunting backdrop for her battle with cancer.

The lockdowns were more than just an inconvenience; they were a suffocating barrier for Andrea. She often reflected on her predicament, wondering how she had found herself in such a dire situation, both physically and emotionally unwell. This chapter of our journey together was just beginning, and I could sense that her story, raw and honest, needed to be told.

Andrea's battle against the odds

The lockdowns in Victoria were a test of endurance for everyone, but they were particularly harrowing for Andrea. With her cancer diagnosis looming over her, the isolation and uncertainty of the pandemic added layers of fear and anxiety to her already overwhelming situation. Despite the grim prognosis, Andrea's resolve to seek alternative healing methods was unwavering.

As the course progressed, we began to connect more deeply, sharing stories and experiences that transcended the classroom. Andrea's journey into natural healing was born out of necessity and a deep-seated belief that there was a better way to approach her health. She immersed herself in research, exploring various holistic treatments and therapies that offered hope where conventional medicine had none.

Her determination was inspiring. Despite the physical toll of her illness and the emotional strain of the lockdowns, Andrea maintained a fierce optimism. She refused to accept her diagnosis as a death sentence and instead viewed it as a challenge to overcome. This resilience was evident in her approach to the course, where she absorbed every bit of knowledge with an admirable and humbling fervor.

Through our conversations, I learned about the profound impact of inflammation on the body and how essential it was to address it for proper healing. This aligned perfectly with my understanding and practice of lymphatic drainage massage. Together, we explored the synergies between our approaches, finding common ground in our shared goal of promoting holistic health.

Andrea's story poignantly reminded us of the human spirit's capacity to fight against the odds. Her journey was not just about battling cancer but about reclaiming her life and health on her terms. It was a testament to the power of belief, perseverance, and the relentless pursuit of healing.

As we neared the end of the course, I felt a deep sense of camaraderie and respect for Andrea. Her story was a beacon of hope for many, a raw and authentic account of a woman who refused to let her circumstances define her.

This chapter of our lives, marked by the shadows of the pandemic and the light of newfound friendships, will forever remain etched in my memory. Our paths intertwined, and we embarked on a mission to bring the healing power of holistic therapy to those who needed it most.

Upon our return to Melbourne, Andrea became very interested in the lymphatic course I was teaching at my clinic once a month. Until now, Andrea has spent a lot of money on Darrell Wolfe's products. They were working to boost her energy and combat the infections ravaging her body, pushing her to the tipping point of her illness. Andrea seemed stuck in the direction of her life—separated, with two teenage boys to raise and a fabulous career in holistic dog teeth grooming. She was excellent at it but struggled to keep a roof over her head with no income during the pandemic, and she felt the isolation of the two years we were ruled, schooled, and fooled.

Andrea struggled with the cost of the products and decided to look for other ways to help her body heal. She loved the lymphatic massage I gave her at Coffs Harbour and noticed a real difference in the fluid retention in her legs. "Wow, I didn't think it would ever go away." Yes, it will—the body is a miracle.

Andrea took my lymphatic drainage course, which changed her life and her approach to health. The SOQI bed stirred up Andrea's energy and health, and in just three intensive days, she saw a remarkable change in her body and mental attitude. And me too—when you have people who support you on every level and don't allow you to fall into limiting belief systems but help you change them— that's the real and raw change we see in people.

Over the coming months, Andrea was in and out of my clinic, using the SOQI bed three times a week. Financially, things were tough for everyone, but I wanted Andrea to use the SOQI bed as often as possible. She found a second-hand SOQI bed for sale at a bargain price and jumped at the chance to invest in her health. Andrea noticed her hair was not falling out, and her energy levels had improved, which provided many other benefits of natural healing.

20   KARA AND ROB

Fifteen years ago, Kara walked into my training studio, her face a canvas of quiet determination and hidden struggle. Diagnosed with Hashimoto's thyroiditis, an autoimmune disorder, Kara also faced iodine deficiency and severe thyroid issues. The thyroid gland, the body's master regulator of metabolism, had become her adversary. She felt perpetually cold despite occasional hot flashes, her hormones a chaotic symphony with no medication to bring them into harmony. A lack of self-confidence compounded Kara's physical challenges. She grappled with side effects from her hypothyroidism medication, which included palpitations, increased appetite, anxiety, weight loss, and insomnia. The toll on her body was evident; she was a slight woman in her late thirties, her frame bearing the marks of her ongoing battle.

When Kara first came to me, I knew little about her struggles. Yet, a beautiful client-teacher friendship blossomed. Kara attended personal training twice weekly, although lifting weights was a monumental task, and cardio seemed impossible. As we worked together, she began to share her life story—years of bullying, few friends, and a pervasive disbelief in her potential. Her long-term partner, Rob, a kind and loving man, was her anchor, helping her find strength when she felt none. Over the years, I witnessed a transformation in Kara. Her confidence grew, as did mine. However, her health continued to decline. She found a fantastic naturopath in Melbourne who started her on a regimen of minerals and vitamins. Initially, it seemed to help, but the reprieve was short-lived. The weight loss persisted, which was a constant concern as I monitored it weekly.

Adding to her woes was a job she despised—a cold, repetitive factory role she'd endured for seven years. Despite these challenges, Kara's resilience shone through. Pilates with me twice weekly transformed Kara into a confident, lovely young lady. This platform has been instrumental in strengthening her core and boosting her confidence. Today, we continue to train together, keeping each other on track. As a trained Pilates instructor, one of my many qualifications, I have seen firsthand the benefits of this practice on mine and my clients' strengths. Kara and I have developed abs of steel thanks to the incredible power of muscle memory at the cellular level. My early years were spent being active, playing sports, and climbing, which laid the foundation for my current strength through this cellular memory.

21   SUE

One day, Andrea, one of my dedicated practitioners, introduced Sue. Little did I know that this meeting would change everything. "Sue, I'm here to help you awaken your body's natural healing power," I said softly, sensing her apprehension. I began the non-surgical treatment, gently working on Sue's shoulder. I reminded her to breathe deeply and relax, guiding her to place her hand gently into the back of her pants to ease the tension and allow me to reach the muscle area of her shoulder blade.

As I worked, I listened intently to her breathing. Something wasn't right; her breaths were labored and sounded more like soft groans. "Sue, how are you feeling?" I asked, my voice laced with concern. There was silence.

"Sue, are you okay?" I repeated, my heart beginning to race. Still no response.

The room seemed to close around us, the air thick with tension. I could feel the hairs on the back of my neck stand up. Something was very wrong.

Sue was a remarkable 38-year-old Asian woman living in Melbourne, Australia. Her journey was one of resilience as she navigated the complex cultural landscape of her adopted home. Despite her warm demeanor and striking features, Sue struggled to find acceptance as an "Aussie" girl. Her story, marked by the challenges of identity and self-acceptance, is a testament to the human spirit's capacity to persevere against all odds.

Sue was undeniably attractive, with a radiant smile and eyes that sparkled with kindness. She carried some weight around her middle, a common trait among many women today. In a world where societal norms often dictate beauty standards, Sue's body became a focal point of her inner conflict. The Western medical community's growing concern over obesity only added to her distress, as doctors emphasized the health risks associated with carrying extra weight.

From a young age, Sue was acutely aware of the societal expectations placed upon her. She had always felt the weight of these literal and metaphorical expectations. The pressure to conform to a specific body image was relentless, and it took a toll on her mental and emotional well-being. Yet, Sue did not shy away from confronting these challenges head-on. She understood that true acceptance had to come from within, not from the validation of others.

In her quest for self-acceptance, Sue often reflected on the broader implications of society's obsession with weight. She pondered why it was so difficult for people to be honest about body image issues. Why couldn't society acknowledge that carrying excess weight was not merely a physical concern but also an emotional and psychological burden? Sue believed that by calling it what it was— fat—people could begin to address the root causes of their struggles with weight and self-image.

Sue's perspective was not rooted in judgment or prejudice. Instead, it stemmed from a place of deep empathy and understanding. She recognized that fear and insecurity had prevented her from confronting the truth about her weight and health. For many, the notion of being labeled "fat" carried a heavy stigma, one that was difficult to shake off. But Sue believed that honesty was the first step toward healing. By accepting the reality of their situation, people could take proactive steps toward improving their health and well-being.

Throughout her journey, Sue encountered women who, like her, were trying to navigate the delicate balance between self-acceptance and societal expectations. Together, they formed a support network, encouraging one another to embrace their bodies and prioritize their health. Sue became a beacon of hope for many, her story resonating with those who felt unseen and unheard in a world that often judged them based on appearances.

Sue's resilience and determination were truly inspiring. Despite the challenges she faced, she never lost sight of her worth. She knew her value was not determined by her weight or ability to conform to societal standards. Instead, her kindness, strength, and unwavering spirit defined her.

"Sue, wake up," I muttered, my heart pounding as dread crept in. Desperation surged, and I called Judy, though mere seconds felt like agonizing minutes. Sue remained unresponsive.

Gently, I lifted her head from the massage chair's face cradle and held it in my hands. Suddenly, a calm and reassuring voice echoed in my mind: "Tap her chest, the middle of her chest bone, to increase the oxygen flow."

I followed the instructions without hesitation. A heartbeat later, Sue's eyes fluttered open. She smiled warmly. "Hi."

Sue was deeply embarrassed; she had soiled her pants. At that moment, Sue had let go of everything. I don't know if Sue stopped breathing or if her heart had stopped; I just don't recall. Sue had a shower; luckily, our clinic has a shower room for clients to use if needed. After 15 minutes in the bathroom, Sue came out and sat down, sharing that she felt fine and was ready to drive home. I asked Sue to stay for another thirty minutes to monitor her and ensure she felt okay.

"What happened?" I asked. "I was only ten minutes into the session, and it seemed like you passed out."

Sue replied, "I don't know. This has never happened before. I was totally fine before I saw you."

Sue left for home, a 45-minute drive away. I asked her to call me when she arrived. The following morning, I spoke to Sue, very concerned.

Sue replied, "I feel like I have been reborn."

"What does that mean?" I wondered.

Sue couldn't believe it or explain it—her pain was gone. It was as if her body had reset. She revisited my clinic two weeks later and booked a non-surgical upper back work session. She was perfectly fine throughout the session.

I asked again, "What happened?"

"I don't know," Sue replied. With her newfound confidence and a different-feeling body, she continued to live life.

Sue's transformation was extraordinary, a testament to the profound healing that can occur when the body is given the proper support. Her story is a beacon of hope for those who have suffered in silence, believing that relief was out of reach. Sue's journey reminds us that miracles can happen, and sometimes, all it takes is a moment of letting go to find a path to renewal and vitality.

22   MICHAEL

Michael was in his late sixties when his daughter, Angela, found me on social media. She had followed my posts for a while and decided to reach out. "Can you help my father? He's been diagnosed with Parkinson's disease," she asked.

I replied, "I'm not sure if I can help, but I can certainly explain how inflammation and stress in his body might be causing symptoms that lead to shaking. If he's willing to hear me out, I'd be happy to try."

Intrigued by this perspective, Angela convinced her father to visit me the following week. Michael walked into my clinic with his wife, Maria, by his side. Michael was not visibly shaking and showed no signs of Parkinson's disease.

I introduced myself and began discussing his health. As I talked to him, I listened to my intuition. "Michael, did you have a traumatic experience as a child? I sense there's something deeply hurting you, causing you great grief."

Michael was taken aback. "I don't know what you mean," he said, but his body language told a different story. His head hung low, his posture closed off, his chest tight. These signs suggested that his upper back was misaligned, restricting the flow of fluid to his brain and potentially causing his tremors.

Michael admitted, "I don't shake all the time. It's only when I'm stressed, but I don't feel stressed. It's strange. My legs stepping forward make me feel unsure of myself, I lack energy and courage."

"Then why are you on medication for Parkinson's?" I asked.

Michael shrugged, "I guess my doctor saw a pattern that fit the disease and thought the medication would help. It doesn't really, but I take it anyway, hoping it might do something."

"Let's see if we can get to the root of this," I said, hopeful that addressing his past trauma and current stress could bring him relief.

Dear Angela,

I saw your dad yesterday for his second session, and he's already feeling better. We've been working on clearing the scar tissue in his back and blocking nerve communication to his legs. Additionally, he was dehydrated, which is affecting his overall well-being.

The root cause, though, is more profound—a lack of self-love and worthiness dates back to his childhood. These suppressed emotions are now surfacing, causing stress and shock-like symptoms that mimic Parkinson's. He's experiencing shaking and uncontrollable movements, but what's happening is a crisis of identity. Your dad is struggling with his sense of manhood, trapped in memories as a way to validate his experiences. This mental and emotional turmoil is leading to a breakdown in his body—oxygen deprivation, cell death, and nerve deterioration, which are reducing his mobility.

This isn't a quick fix. While Michael feels excellent after two sessions, we must continue clearing these deep-seated issues from his tissues. This process involves the lymphatic system draining toxins and emotional blockages.

I encouraged Mary to schedule another appointment for him. I understand how busy life can be, yet what could be more important than healing? Running around takes a toll, but healing can give him the strength and vitality to live more fully. Let's prioritize his health and well-being.

Hi Michelle,
He is doing well. We went to Italy for three weeks; Michael could walk everywhere and do anything! Thank you so much! Michael loved and appreciated the message. I will ask them if I can encourage them to make another appointment. Yes, lots more work is needed.
xxx

The echoes of the past

After the session with Michael and Maria, I felt emotion wash over me. I held back the tears, my heart heavy with the weight of Michael's unspoken pain. I had been trying to help Michael understand that the agony in his body was deeply rooted in the memories of his childhood.

Growing up in a boarding school in the fifties had been brutal and uncompromising. As a young boy, Michael had felt unwanted, abandoned by his parents, and deprived of love. This was not true, but from a young boy's perspective, it was. These feelings of abandonment and grief had etched themselves into his cellular memory, buried deep within him for decades. They were a silent burden, growing increasingly unbearable over time, yet only Michael could hear their cry.

These memories shocked his body, causing it to react beyond his control. Michael experienced relentless shaking, dehydration, joint stiffness, pain, disrupted sleep, exhaustion, and an inability to breathe deeply. The stress had wreaked havoc on his nervous system, leading to inflammation that crystallized and blocked the flow of oxygen to his spine and brain.

As I explained this to Michael, he looked at me wide-eyed. "Wow," he said, his voice filled with awe and understanding.

Maria, too, was overwhelmed. "Oh, my goodness," she exclaimed. "I knew all along, but no-one ever listened to me."

Michael didn't return for another appointment; maybe he didn't need to.

23   GIUSEPPE

A transformative encounter

In 2023, I embarked on a transformative journey in Coffs Harbour, a serene coastal town. There, while attending a Non-Surgical Health

Course, I encountered Giuseppe. Our first challenge was the Life Coach Course, designed to shatter the core of our belief systems and rewire our minds.

The course's approach was as unconventional as it was powerful: "crack everyone's coconut." This vivid metaphor aptly describes breaking open entrenched belief systems and exposing the underlying mechanisms governing our lives. It was an eye-opening way to reveal the subconscious programs that dictate our actions, often without us even realizing it.

The dynamic among the participants was compelling: five men and twenty women, all drawn together by a shared desire for profound change. The 12-day course was intense and immersive, structured to make us confront and unravel the internal scripts that silently directed our lives.

As we dove more deeply, the intensity grew. We were forced to face our deepest fears, challenge our most ingrained beliefs, and recognize the invisible programs running our lives. The experience was daunting and exhilarating, pushing us to the brink and guiding us towards breakthroughs.

It's crucial to recognize when a man is uncertain and feeling vulnerable to understand and help him cope with his emotions. Take Giuseppe, a gentleman in his fifties who wanted to change his life and believed this was the place to do it. Giuseppe was quiet, often sitting at the back, unsure whether to speak up or remain silent.

He had been raised in a traditional Italian culture with strong family connections, yet for now, Giuseppe's life had taken a different turn. His once firm belief in family unity had shattered long ago, with his daughter no longer speaking to him and a marriage that had fallen apart. He was left feeling very lonely. Giuseppe was lost in a world of pain, although he didn't initially attribute this to his heart attack a few years ago. The emotional strain had taken its toll, and now he searched for answers without knowing what he was looking for.

For many people, this search often boils down to seeking love—love for oneself, love in a partner, and love for one's children, regardless of age. Giuseppe's journey was about finding that love and healing the deep emotional wounds he carried.

I had often observed Giuseppe from afar. Something about him drew people in: an air of quiet resilience. One day, as a group of us were chatting, Giuseppe approached me with a curious glint in his eye.

"Can you help me?" he asked, eager to learn more about my background and the mysterious practice of lymphatic drainage. Intrigued by the potential benefits, he wanted to understand how it could aid healing.

That afternoon, Giuseppe booked a session with me. I could sense his tension and the weight of untold stories as he lay on the table. With each gentle touch, I could feel him relaxing, his barriers slowly crumbling. During this session, Giuseppe found a semblance of peace for the first time in what felt like forever. He began sharing his story in a voice tinged with relief and vulnerability. Opening up to a stranger is no small feat; it requires immense courage. But this moment was a turning point for him, a step towards healing.

After the session, Giuseppe sat up, his face filled with amazement. "How do you do that?" he asked, his voice filled with wonder.

With a smile, I replied, "It takes practice, like anything in life. From humble beginnings to a deep understanding of the innate intelligence within us all."

In the following days, Giuseppe and I worked together to create a six-month program for him. We set small, achievable goals to guide him from the start date to the finish line. This plan was designed, not just for healing, but for transformation.

Giuseppe's journey had begun, and I was honored to be a part of it. Little did I know, this experience would also deepen my understanding of the profound impact of lymphatic drainage, reinforcing my belief in its power to heal and transform lives.

A few months later, I called Giuseppe to check if he had followed his plan. To my disappointment, he had not started working on his goals. His health had deteriorated further, and he was suffering from severe knee pain without understanding the cause. I know from experience that if you don't follow your path here on earth, your innate intelligence will keep presenting you with life experiences until you do, but Giuseppe wasn't listening.

24   ELLEN

Judy accompanied me on a home visit in Melbourne's eastern suburbs, where we were scheduled to provide a 90-minute lymphatic drainage massage. Our patient, Ellen, was an elderly lady in her seventies who struggled with heavy, swollen legs and used a stick for support. The house was old, musty, and dimly lit, with a flickering gas fire casting sporadic light. Ellen sat in a rocking chair, her legs visibly swollen and reddened. Her midsection was hard as a rock, a condition that contributed to severe fluid retention, causing her ankles and feet to swell so much that her toes were almost invisible.

Ellen's condition began when she started a medication regimen for epilepsy at just 12 years old. Ellen explained to me it was just after her first monthly cycle, and she thought she was crazy with blood and went into a meltdown of fits. She experienced extreme anxiety due to her bleeding, causing her body to become uncontrollably tense with worry. This nervous tension was initially mistaken for epilepsy by doctors, and she had been on medication ever since.

This marked the start of a downward spiral in her health, though Ellen didn't fully realize its extent at the time.

I decided to begin the treatment by using the E-power device on Ellen's legs to energize her cells, allowing oxygen to penetrate and break up calcification through the frequency belt. Starting on her right side, I applied firm pressure, careful not to cause pain. Ellen immediately noticed a difference, saying it felt unlike any other lymphatic massage she had experienced. Her feet began to soften, and sensation returned to her legs and feet.

Ellen mentioned that she had used compression pumps on her legs that morning but that felt ineffective. I explained that while compression pumps might aid in circulation, they only treat a part of the body rather than the whole. True healing comes from hands-on techniques that generate the necessary electrical impulses for proper blood flow, not from wrapping legs in plastic and turning on a machine.

Ellen was surprised to feel so much better after such a short time. She then shared her life story with me. She had been on a relentless cycle of medication and surgeries, managing illness after illness. Despite all her efforts, she ended up with a massive bag of pills and numerous side effects, including significant weight gain—25 kilos in just twelve months. Ellen was determined not to succumb to the same fate as her family: her husband had died of cancer, her sister had heart disease, and even her daughter was struggling with multiple surgeries and health conditions.

Ellen's resilience and determination to improve her health were inspiring. She was committed to walking again and breaking free from the cycle of illness that had plagued her family. Our session marked the beginning of a new chapter for her as she took control of her health and sought treatments that addressed her body as a whole. I don't know if I'll see her again. Ellen walked Judy and me to the door, surprised that she was walking better and her legs felt lighter. We said our goodbyes, wishing her the best of luck.

25 NICOLE

A glimmer of hope

Nicole walked into my clinic with her shoulders sagging under despair, tears barely concealed behind a brave facade. She had just reached breaking point, falling to her knees in desperation and praying for help. In a moment of clarity, she turned to Google and found my website. As she read through my information, a spark of hope ignited within her. "I knew it," she whispered to herself, "there is an answer for fluid retention, for edema."

Nicole's journey had been long and arduous. Twenty-five years ago, she had battled breast cancer, that resulted in a double mastectomy. This left a deep emotional scar, a constant reminder of her pain every time she looked in the mirror. She felt a profound loss of her womanhood, a feeling that haunted her daily. Her story was one of resilience and heartache, the details of which I am to keep confidential. Yet, an event from when she was sixteen had fuelled her determination to overcome her health challenges.

Nicole's body had been swelling uncontrollably, and no-one had been able to provide her with answers or relief. This results from a severely blocked lymphatic system, causing a backup of fluid called stress and inflammation within the body.

Doctors had told her there was no cure for her condition. "Do you believe that you'll live in this body you despise forever?" I asked her gently.

Nicole looked at me with sorrow-filled eyes and shook her head. "No," she replied, "there has to be a way to reverse these symptoms."

"Yes," I said, "there is. But I can't do it alone. You'll have to find the answers you seek, and I can help you along the way."

In her first session, we began with an energy bed treatment and a thirty-minute lymphatic drainage massage. Nicole felt an immediate connection to the process. She was hooked and booked a package of ten sessions. Nicole shared her ambitious goal with me: "I am on a mission to lose weight, eliminate all my fluid retention, and fit into a swimsuit for my holiday in June this year. Let's make it happen." Nicole had previously invested in expensive compression pumps for her legs, which were uncomfortable and ineffective. After her first session with me, she put those pumps away for good.

It would be a transformative journey to restore Nicole's body to where she wanted it to be. I saw her every week for a ninety-minute session. During these sessions, we delved into the deep emotional feelings that surfaced. Nicole was often astonished by the questions I posed. "How did you know that?" she would ask, wide-eyed.

I would simply smile and say, "It's just something I do."

In one session, I sensed a profound emotional turmoil that had plagued her for most of her life. "This unresolved pain," I said gently, "has been a significant contributor to your illness and has hindered your path to health and wellness."

Nicole, taken aback, took a deep breath and hesitated before speaking. "I've never told anyone this except my husband," she said slowly. "He knows, but no-one else does."

She then shared with me, over the next twenty minutes, the harrowing experience she endured as a young teenager. The pain lingered, unresolved and festering, impacting her life continuously.

Nicole's journey led her into a career where she could exert control over men, an unusual move but the only way she felt she could thrive in a male-dominated world. By being the boss, she found her role in life. However, this came with emotional suppression that Nicole didn't understand until I helped her see what was happening. She was surprised but also recognized that her behavior was a defense mechanism. She was shielding herself from the indescribable pain she experienced during her early teenage years.

With each session, Nicole made remarkable progress. She began losing weight, and I was finally able to massage areas that were previously off-limits, like her breast area. Although Nicole initially felt disgusted, she started seeing the light. Nicole grew increasingly confident about her upcoming flight overseas as her holiday approached. No more leg compressions, no more fluid retention—she felt terrific. After eight months of dedicated work, Nicole experienced a new lease on life. She committed to exercising daily, feeling empowered and energized instead of slow and weighed down by fluid retention.

When the time came to fly across the seas for her beautiful trip with her family, Nicole embraced her new life at 54 with confidence and joy, ready to enjoy her holiday in her new bathing suit.

26   KATE

The lesson of Kate

People come into our lives to teach us something every day, often unexpectedly. Kate was a new client who walked into my clinic one day, and I had a feeling I wouldn't see her again after that session. She entered with a sorrowful energy as if she carried the world's weight on her shoulders. Young and seemingly burdened, Kate shared her story with me, painting a picture of a life filled with challenges.

Kate was a single mother of three children—eleven, eight, and two years old. She homeschooled them, a task demanding immense patience and energy. Yet, Kate struggled with a pervasive darkness that seemed to cloud her every moment. Despite her faith—she was a devout Christian who followed the light of freedom—Kate had fallen into a deep, dark place. Kate needed a kind heart to help her return to the light.

As we spoke, it became clear that Kate was a beautiful soul with so much to give, yet she had neglected to take care of herself. She found solace in our clinic, a calmness that she desperately needed. She discovered a newfound peace she had been searching for in that space. Kate confided in me that she didn't have many friends. I explained that as Kate grew and evolved, she often outpaced her friends, reaching levels of understanding and experience that even Kate struggled to comprehend.

As Kate left after our session, I pondered the nature of life and relationships. It struck me how amazing it is that we constantly learn and grow through the people we meet. Kate's visit reminded me of my journey and the people who had left my life. I realized that, just like Kate, I had seen people leave my life as quickly as they had entered it, even those I thought would be with me forever.

Growth is a personal journey; sometimes, the people around us don't grow simultaneously. It's okay to let them go. Kate's lesson in my life was clear. As we evolve, it's natural for some relationships to fall away. The key is to cherish the moments we share, learn from them, and move forward with an open heart, ready to embrace life's next lesson.

Kate's story reminds us that we all have the power to find light in our darkest times, often through the kindness and support of others. As we continue to grow, we must remember that it's okay to outgrow relationships. Every person we meet brings a lesson, and every lesson brings us closer to our true selves.

27   GUNDA

The unlikely encounter

Gunda had been Christopher's loyal client for many years, frequenting his hairdressing salon that buzzed with life at the front of the clinic. Christopher, a man of many talents, had a dual role: styling hair and managing the bustling salon while promoting the hidden gem at the back of the shop, Lymphology Australia.

Gunda, a woman of curiosity and skepticism, was increasingly intrigued by the mysterious business behind the salon. Despite

Christopher's best attempts to explain the transformative therapy offered by Lymphology Australia, Gunda remained uncertain but deeply curious. One day, her curiosity overcame her hesitation, and she decided to discover more.

Gunda was carrying a heavy burden. The weight and pain in her legs were debilitating, rendering her days long and arduous. Each step felt like she was dragging tree branches, and the relentless discomfort took a toll on her once vibrant spirit. Gunda intensely disliked doctors and specialists, viewing them as harbingers of empty promises and cold, sterile solutions. She had sought answers for her condition but found none, leaving her disillusioned and despairing.

Gunda lived alone and cherished her independence. She had no husband or children but enjoyed a rich social life filled with friends and outings. However, her legs were betraying her, limiting her mobility and dampening her joy. She resented the thought of slowing down and felt trapped in a body that was failing her.

When Gunda finally met me, she was skeptical. As we sat down to discuss her condition, she voiced her doubts. "I hate exercise," she admitted, her eyes filled with frustration, "and I don't see how anything can change this."

I understood her reluctance and explained, "Give us one chance, Gunda. Just one session to see if we can make a difference."

She hesitated, her skepticism battling with a glimmer of hope. Gunda's life had been marked by resilience and independence, and the thought of finding relief, even from an unconventional source, was a beacon in her darkening world. She agreed to try if only to prove her doubts right.

That first session was transformative. Gunda felt a lightness she hadn't experienced in years. The pain in her legs began to alleviate, replaced by a newfound energy. She was astonished by the immediate results and found herself eager for more sessions. Each visit brought further improvement, and slowly, the weight in her legs lifted, freeing her from the prison of pain she had been trapped in for so long.

Gunda's transformation was nothing short of miraculous. She regained her mobility and zest for life, embracing her social activities with renewed vigor. Her skepticism melted away, replaced by gratitude and belief in the healing power of Lymphology Australia.

Her story became a testament to the clinic's potential, and Gunda, once a doubter, became one of its most passionate advocates. Her journey from pain to freedom inspired many, showcasing the extraordinary impact of this miracle therapy hidden behind a bustling hairdressing salon.

28   DAVID

Overcoming the pain

It was a brisk October morning when I received an unexpected phone call from a lovely lady named Nicki. Her voice carried a mix of hope and urgency, a combination I was all too familiar with in my work. To my surprise, Nicki had met Sean—another Lymphologist who is now a well-known lymphatic drainage practitioner—many years ago. Nicki sought my help for her husband, David, who was facing a scheduled complete knee replacement in early January 2024. As we spoke, Nicki expressed her concerns about David's severe knee pain and the impending surgery. She asked if I could help him. I explained that we had two options: we could work to avoid the knee replacement surgery altogether or prepare his knee to ensure the operation would be less painful and the recovery quicker. Either way, I was confident I could significantly improve David's condition.

The following week, David made an appointment to see me. He was eager, yet cautious, his curiosity piqued by the prospect of finally alleviating the pain that had plagued him for decades. His knee injury, a relic from his football days 40 years ago, had grown worse over time. To complicate matters, he had undergone surgery on his other knee just a year or two ago, and the recovery had been long and arduous. David wasn't looking forward to another round of surgery, but was desperate to return to competitive tennis, and to live without the constant pain that came with every movement.

During our initial consultation, we set a comprehensive plan in motion. We aimed to reduce pain, restore mobility in both knees and reclaim his active lifestyle. David's determination was palpable, fuelled by his longing to play tennis and move freely again. As we embarked on this journey together, I couldn't help but feel a sense of purpose and anticipation. This endeavor was more than just a medical intervention; it was a testament to the resilience of the human spirit and the transformative power of healing. David came to see me twice a week for the first four weeks. During our initial consultation, I mentioned a non-surgical session to break down the scar tissue blocking his knee's mechanics. David was a real estate broker, a high-pressure job that had kept him under constant stress for 35 years. Stress had been his fuel, pushing him through each day, but it had taken a toll on his body. He was now paying the price with diabetes, high blood pressure, and a large waistline.

Non-surgical sessions are genuinely transformative. For healing to occur, we need to convert scar tissue back into connective tissue, dissolve crystallization, and relocate displaced calcium back to the bones. This approach can remarkably restore bones to a healthy condition, regardless of the patient's age, by gently separating the fibers that hinder the body's natural healing process. With this, we embarked on a 12-month plan to regenerate David's body.

The first two sessions of non-surgical treatment were incredibly successful. David couldn't believe it—he was now doing more with his knees than he had in years and without pain. How could this be? The transformation had begun. Next was David's extensive waste line non-surgical abdominal lift.

Again, David was surprised by the quick result of being less tired, having more energy and a shrinking waistline. I mentioned to him that it was his medication causing all his issues and that his eating habits could be better, but overall, David's eating habits weren't bad. We must understand anything foreign to our system the body gets rid of as waste, and believe it or not, this is 98 percent of what we eat. I asked David if he could discuss with his doctors to reduce the medication, and David said he would.

David visited his Endocrinologist. Endocrinologists specialize in the endocrine system, which includes glands and hormones. They often manage conditions like diabetes, thyroid disorders, and other metabolic issues. She told him that he must stay on his medication. That said, I continued doing my best with David's program.

Three months into his healing journey, David canceled his knee surgery. His specialist said, "We will be here if you need us down the track." David felt great physically and mentally and was thrilled to have found a path to wellness that didn't involve going under the knife. His doctors, while supportive, suggested they could always reschedule the surgery if needed. However, life was looking up for David, and he was determined to continue his recovery naturally.

Then, one day at home, everything changed. As he walked down the hallway, he tripped over his dog, and before he knew it, he was on the floor, his knee throbbing in excruciating pain. He was furious with himself—how could he be so careless? The incident shook his confidence, and by the week's end, he reconsidered his decision. Maybe surgery was the right choice after all.

After discussing it with his specialist, David reluctantly proceeded with the operation. Determined to ensure the best possible outcome, I designed a specialized program to strengthen the muscles around his knee, aiming to reduce his recovery time and minimize post-operative pain. The surgery day arrived, and the operation was deemed a success—until the surgeons informed him they had accidentally nicked a nerve. David developed a drop foot, making it difficult to lift his foot, and he was now struggling with stiffness in his new knee.

David was left questioning everything—had he made the right decision?

We worked on his ankle non-surgically, which resulted in faster foot healing and a great outcome in David's recovery.

29   SUE

A journey begins

Sue was a beautiful soul trapped in a body that betrayed her. For forty long years, her knees and back had been a source of relentless agony, a pain that no treatment, therapy, or medication seemed able to alleviate. Seventy-nine years old, Sue had grown accustomed to the ache, a constant, unwelcome companion in her daily life. Her spirit, however, remained unbroken. She was yearning for a respite she had long thought impossible.

I don't know how Sue came to see me. She was a stranger until the day she walked into my practice, accompanied by Naomi, a kind-hearted caregiver who had been looking after her. Naomi had heard about lymphatic drainage and its potential to ease bodily pain. Though she couldn't fully explain the process, she hoped it might offer Sue some relief.

Sue and I sat down to discuss her condition. She had been on antidepressant drugs for forty years, a testament to the weight of her suffering. She felt heavy, not just in her body but in her soul, burdened by decades of unrelenting pain. Despite this, Sue wasn't ready to give up on life. Her determination to find some measure of comfort was palpable.

Naomi, ever the optimist, suggested that lymphatic drainage might be beneficial. Sue looked at her with a mix of skepticism and hope. "What's that?" she asked, her voice tinged with curiosity.

Naomi shrugged, offering a gentle smile. "I've heard great things about it. They say it can reduce pain in the body. Even if it's just a massage, it might do you some good."

Sue nodded slowly, a glimmer of hope flickering in her eyes. "Okay," she said, "we shall go. Even if it's just a massage, it will be good."

And so, her journey began. It was a journey of hope, healing, and discovering something that would change Sue's life forever. This story is about how Sue found relief and how a seemingly simple treatment transformed her body and entire existence. Sue was a woman who had dedicated much of her life to her community, always putting others' needs before her own. But now, she found herself in need of healing and relief. The pain and weight she carried were not just physical but deeply emotional, rooted in years of struggle and sacrifice.

Her carer Naomi, who had seen the toll it had taken on her, recommended a session with a SOQI bed and a Chi machine. Sue, always open to new experiences, agreed to try it.

The SOQI bed, with its three heat domes, enveloped Sue in a warm embrace, increasing the oxygen in her body and boosting her immunity. As the gentle heat seeped into her muscles, she felt a soothing calmness wash over her, a peace she hadn't felt in years. The Chi machine's gentle rocking provided a subtle body alignment, relaxing her tight muscles and strengthening the weakened ones. For 30 minutes, she lay there, feeling the gentle massage and the warmth cocooning her, a profound sense of tranquillity settling in her soul.

After the session, Sue was astonished at how good she felt. The pain that had been her constant companion was now a distant memory. Naomi was thrilled with the outcome, knowing how much Sue did for others and how desperately she needed this relief.

Sue had already lost considerable weight but had hit a plateau. During a conversation, I mentioned to her that the medication she was on might be contributing to her inability to lose more weight. "Perhaps you could discuss with your doctor the possibility of gradually reducing your medication," I suggested.

Taking this advice to heart, Sue visited her doctor and explained her new regimen and her remarkable improvement. To her delight, the doctor was supportive. "If you're feeling this good, Sue, we can consider tapering off your medication, even your antidepressants," he said.

Sue was overjoyed. She embarked on a new journey, one that didn't rely on pills but on natural healing and self-care. As she slowly weaned off her medication, the weight began to melt away. But the most complex challenge remained: her lifelong reliance on sugary foods to fill the void in her lonely heart and soothe her emotional trauma.

Living with her oldest daughter under one roof added another layer of complexity to her struggle. Their relationship was strained, and the emotional tension often led Sue to seek comfort in sweets. But now, with her newfound strength and determination, Sue was ready to face these challenges head-on.

Through perseverance and support, Sue began to overcome her dependency on sugar. She found healthier ways to cope with her emotions and rebuild her relationship with her daughter. The journey was difficult, but Sue's unwavering resolve and the support of those around her made all the difference.

In the end, Sue's story is one of incredible transformation. She not only shed the physical weight but also the emotional burdens that had held her back for so long. Her healing journey was a testament to the power of natural therapies, the importance of support, and the incredible strength of the human spirit.

Sue's experience with the SOQI bed and Chi machine began a new chapter in her life, one filled with hope, health, and happiness. She became an inspiration to her community, showing that with the right tools and mindset, anyone can overcome their challenges and find their path to wellness.

Sue's own words

Hi everyone, I just want to share my journey with Michelle. Around this time last year in 2023, I developed pain in my whole body; doctors said it was arthritis. I found it hard to walk and do all the things I needed to do around the house and in the garden, as I had lost my husband to bone cancer in July 2021. My daughter was moving in with me at the time, and she had a social worker helping her, so she decided to help me, taking me to doctors, who and only prescribed Panadol Osteo twice a day. That didn't do anything to stop the pain. Then, one day, she somehow found Michelle and took me to see her. I was 92 kg— and trying to stay happy, which is not easy when you are in pain. I had never experienced having a caring person massaging me, let alone going on an energy bed, that made my ankles wobble, but Michelle was so encouraging and got me talking about my past life experiences.

She began to teach me about letting go of past hurts, etc., and to be happy, explaining how I had gut problems and inflammation that was affecting my health. Michelle helped me to learn to eat unprocessed food and more veggies, go gluten-free and stop the sugar which she said was poison to my body and to have the special drops she gave me. After a few weeks, I found that I had lost 12 kg. She was doing non-surgical treatments on me; she would, for instance, put her elbow on the side of my knee and push real hard, telling me to breathe while she counted to ten. It hurt like crazy, but it was worth it; no more knee pain, woohoo! I was on antidepressants at the time, which I was encouraged to give up, and I have done slowly. I am now in the process of giving up other medications I am taking for high blood pressure, Somac tablet for Hiatus hernia, and Thyroid tablet. I think I inherited anxiety from my mum, so I have rescue remedy lollies that help heaps. I also have herbal digestive lollies that help.

30　KAITLIN

Kaitlin walked into my office, frail and softly spoken, her presence a heart-wrenching sight. Diagnosed with a rare and aggressive cancer, she had endured a whirlwind of medical interventions, including the removal of her ovaries and both breasts just twelve months ago. A highly educated woman, Kaitlin was determined to finish her PhD in geology, a pursuit she had begun many years prior. She had a loving husband and two young boys who were the center of her world.

Her intelligent mind grappled with the cruel reality of her health. At that moment, I found myself at a loss for words, which rarely happens to me. I simply listened, knowing that was the most precious gift I could offer her. Her pain was beyond comprehension, a hundred out of ten. The medication meant to alleviate her suffering often caused her more agony than the cancer itself. For six months, she was confined to her home, battling incessant, debilitating symptoms.

Yet, despite her exhaustion, she was determined to finish her PhD and see her sons grow up. Kaitlin sought my help for severe fluid retention in her right arm, which had become so swollen that she could no longer write. After just one session of lymphatic drainage massage, her pain was halved, offering her a fleeting moment of relief in an otherwise relentless ordeal. Kaitlin scheduled another appointment, but I knew this small respite wouldn't change the trajectory of her life. It was merely a moment of comfort from a stranger. As she lay on the massage table, too sore to move, holding back tears, she reminded me of my sister Julie during her cancer journey—pale, with little circulation and a low oxygen count. Kaitlin remained very still, absorbing the tender touch of a stranger. In her gentle voice, she confided, "Michelle, I wish I could stop my medication; the pain it causes is unbearable. But they say I could possibly live another year, and for the chance to see my boys grow a little more, I will endure this for them." On Wednesday, August 7th, 2024, my heart silently screamed,

"Oh my Lord..." Kaitlin was only 32 years old.

31   VICTOR

Victor had always dreamed of returning home to Egypt, but his failing health kept him grounded, thousands of miles away from the place that held his heart. A broken man with a heart sustained by a pacemaker, Victor's journey was one of desperation. For 72 years, he had been starved of love—not just from others, but from himself. His heart, encased in a fortress of sorrow, struggled to beat, suffocating from the weight of unhealed wounds.

Victor's search for salvation led him to me. After finding my name on Google, we spoke at length about his condition. I assured him that anything could be changed, that his body, though deprived of oxygen and burdened by heartache, was not beyond repair. His heart, dependent on a pacemaker to regulate its rhythm, was a testament to his lifelong struggle—a struggle that began with a deep, unfulfilled longing for love.

The pacemaker, a small device implanted under the skin, sent electrical signals to keep Victor's heart beating. But no device could mend a heart broken by decades of emotional pain. Victor tried to fill the void with material things, believing love could be bought. But this only led him further into darkness, ensnaring him in relationships that fed his despair rather than his soul.

When Victor arrived for his session, his body reflected the turmoil within. His stomach was enormous, a glaring symptom of the imbalance that plagued him. We began with a session in the SOQI bed, followed by 30 minutes of lymphatic drainage massage. His body, desperately dehydrated and mechanically inefficient, needed to be restored. The healing journey required breaking down of the physical barriers that trapped him in his suffering.

Yet, despite everything, Victor's spirit clung to a profound understanding: that the body, crafted in God's image, held an infinite capacity for healing. But life had been unkind, and the people closest to him had shattered his faith, leaving him on the brink of surrender. His heart was shut down, his mind clouded, and his spirit lost in a labyrinth of despair.

But a spark of hope began to flicker in that moment of darkness. Through our work together, Victor started to see the possibility of redemption. His journey was far from over, but he no longer walked alone. With each session, his body grew stronger, his heart began to heal, and the path back to Egypt, once obscured by illness and doubt, became more evident.

Victor stepped into the clinic with an energy that was impossible to ignore. Just four days ago, he had arrived burdened with the weight of years of struggle and heartache, his body and spirit exhausted from the relentless trial life had thrown his way. But today, he was a different man. The transformation was as clear as the broad smile that now graced his face, a smile that hadn't seen the light of day for years.

As Victor approached, I noticed a familiar glint in his eyes, a spark of vitality absent during our first meeting. He held a piece of paper, folded neatly, almost reverently. As he drew closer, I could see it was a report from his doctor. He handed it to me with a particular pride, a subtle but profound gesture that spoke volumes.

"Well done," were the words scrawled across the top of the report in the doctor's handwriting. But those two simple words carried the weight of a lifetime of struggle and the beginning of a new chapter for Victor.

Without hesitation, he gently wrapped his arms around me in a hug. It was a hug filled with gratitude, hope, and peace. "Wow," he whispered, as if unable to fully grasp the enormity of his feelings, "I've booked my flight back home."

Victor paused, letting those words settle into the space between us. Then, with his voice trembling slightly with emotion, he added, "For the first time in years, I feel alive. My heart is mending."

I stood there, holding that moment close, knowing this was more than just a routine check-up or a mere update from a patient. This moment was the culmination of Victor's journey back to himself, which had taken him across continents, through the corridors of hospitals, and into the depths of his soul. His words resonated deeply, not just because they signaled a physical healing, but because they spoke to something far more significant—healing the heart, the spirit, and the very essence of who he was.

Victor's story had always been one of resilience and quiet determination. Victor had faced heartache for 72 long years, each beat of his heart a reminder of the trials he had endured. His pacemaker had become a symbol of his struggle, managing the electrical currents that kept him alive but not truly living. It was as if he had been merely existing, trapped in a body that no longer felt like his own.

But something had shifted in those four days since I last saw him. The work we had done together—utilizing the SOQI bed, lymphatic drainage massage, and other non-surgical therapies—had begun to rehydrate his body and spirit. It was as if the parched soil of his soul had finally found the water it so desperately needed, allowing life to bloom once more.

Victor had always believed, on some level, in the body's ability to heal, but that belief had been tested time and again by the harsh realities of his condition. And yet, despite everything, he had never completely lost hope. That hope, fragile as it had been, was now a roaring flame within him, fuelled by his progress.

Looking at him, I could see the outlines of a man who had redis-covered his health and purpose. His decision to return to Egypt was more than just a geographical move; it was a return to the life he had longed for, a life that had seemed so far out of reach for so long.

The Victor standing before me was no longer the weary, defeated man who had walked into my clinic just days before. He was a man reborn, with a heart that was mending, not just physically, but emotionally and spiritually as well. The years of heartache had left their mark, but they had also forged a strength within him that was now shining through, carrying him forward into this new chapter of his life.

As Victor left the clinic that day, I felt a deep sense of fulfill-ment. His journey had become a part of my own, a testament to the incredible power of the human spirit and the body's innate ability to heal when given the right tools and support. His story was far from over, but this chapter ended with a victory that was nothing short of miraculous.

Victor's flight home was booked, and with it, he carried not just his belongings, but a heart full of hope—a heart that was finally beginning to heal. As he walked away, I knew that the Victor I had come to know and care for would not just survive—he would thrive.

32   KAREN

Karen and her daughter – life lessons

Karen, a fifty-seven-year-old woman, felt adrift in a foreign and confusing world. She was unaware of how lost she was, navigating life with the best intentions but without a clear direction. Her heart ached for understanding, not just for herself but also for her daughter, who was teetering on the edge of adolescence, searching for something she couldn't grasp.

Karen had heard whispers about my ability to help teenagers find their way back to themselves, to rediscover the light within that had dimmed under the pressures of life. Desperate and hopeful, she booked an appointment for her daughter, hoping that somehow, through me, they could both find the clarity they desperately needed.

When they arrived, I could see they were more alike than they realized—two peas in a pod, silently screaming for understanding, for someone to hear the unspoken words buried deep within their hearts. Karen sat outside the room, her hands tightly clasped in her lap, as I spoke with her daughter. The young girl, hesitant at first, began to open up, her emotions spilling over like a dam breaking after years of holding back.

As she spoke, it became clear that it was Karen, not her daughter, who had truly been seeking help all along. The words that tumbled out were not just her daughter's, but Karen's silent pleas for guidance for a path forward in a world that had become too overwhelming to navigate alone. Her daughter had booked a session the following week. I went out to greet them, but it was only Karen.

Karen was a devoted mother who always put her daughter first, yet she felt burdened by the world's weight. Struggling to lose weight and unaware of the emotional toll she was taking, Karen sought something to help her feel better. That's when she decided to try the SOQI bed and lymphatic massage.

Karen's daughter was a high achiever, constantly striving for approval, and Karen couldn't shake her concern and fear for her. One day, I told Karen, "You're looking into a mirror."

My words left her silent momentarily, and then she finally admitted, "Yes, I didn't want to see it."

"How could I have missed this?" she asked, grappling with the realization. It's a million-dollar question. When you're trapped in your own limiting beliefs and emotional baggage, it's hard to see anything.

Karen's daughter left for Europe the following week, marking the beginning of Karen's journey of self-discovery. At fifty-seven, she looked deeply at herself for the first time and didn't like what she saw. After five sessions of emotional clearing, Karen realized that she was full of anxiety, fear, and worry—traits that had plagued her throughout her life.

Karen came from a family of Holocaust survivors, and as a child, she had lived through those stories told by her mother. She carried the burden of that traumatic history, which manifested as what I call "issues on your tissues." These unresolved emotions haunted Karen, making her jumpy and fearful without apparent reason.

By confronting these deep-seated issues, Karen began to heal, shedding the generational weight holding her back. Her transformation story shows that it's never too late to look inward, face the truth, and reclaim your life.

33   NAEEMA

A call for healing

The phone rang, shattering the stillness of the afternoon. As I picked it up, I could hear the tremor in her voice—Naeema, a young mother of five, was on the other end, desperate and in agony. At only 32, her body had borne the brunt of three C-sections, and now, after her fifth child, her midsection was in turmoil. Her muscles were weak, and there had been no time for recovery.

But it wasn't just the exhaustion of motherhood that had pushed Naeema to her breaking point. A lump had started to form near her belly button, it was growing rapidly and causing excruciating pain. The doctors had convinced her that surgery was the only option. They told her it was likely scar tissue pushing up from her large intestines, but their solution—a mesh implanted beneath her belly button—only seemed to make things worse.

"Wire, really?" I exclaimed, shocked. "Bloody hell, that's a new one."

Naeema's pain had reached a crescendo, leaving her unable to focus on her children, her life, or even her will to go on. She felt as if life was slipping through her fingers, leaving behind only the unbearable ache in her body.

Desperate and broken, Naeema fell to her knees and prayed for an answer to her suffering. In that moment of raw vulnerability, she found a sliver of hope. I could sense it over the phone, a spark that needed nurturing.

I spoke to her with warmth and conviction, the conviction that comes from knowing the body's incredible capacity for healing. "You must believe," I told her gently. The body can do so much more than we give it credit for. We just need to give it a chance."

My words resonated with her, giving her the courage to take the next step. By the end of the call, Naeema had made up her mind. She booked an appointment to see me the next day, ready to embark on a healing journey that would change her life forever.

Naeema walked into my practice, burdened by the weight of years of struggle, both physically and emotionally. Her petite frame was carrying far too much weight, a reminder of her five pregnancies and the toll they had taken on her body. She was determined to reclaim her pre-pregnancy body, a goal that felt just out of reach despite her best efforts with diet and exercise.

Naeema had grown weary of the medication she had been prescribed, understanding that it was only adding to the heaviness she felt within. She had done her research and uncovered the troubling side effects of the drugs. She was resolute in her decision to find a natural path to healing.

Our first session was transformative. As I worked on her waistline, gently stimulating her lymphatic system and reintroducing oxygen into her tissues, something remarkable happened—Naeema's pain, which had been her constant companion, simply vanished. She left that day feeling lighter, almost as if a burden had been lifted from her shoulders.

I suggested she return the following week to see how her body responded. When she walked in a week later, her face was radiant, and she greeted me with the biggest hug. "I don't know what you did," she said, her voice filled with gratitude, "but I am pain-free now. I have a new energy and a love for life I thought I'd lost."

With her newfound vitality, Naeema began to turn her life around. She embraced her role as a mother of six with renewed joy and purpose, finding time for herself amid her busy life. Naeema continues to see me whenever she can, and her story is a testament to the power of hope and the incredible ability of the body to regenerate and heal when given the proper support.

34   VANESSA

The power of healing

The air buzzed with energy as I entered the room at an event where healthcare professionals from various fields gathered to share their expertise. I had been invited to speak about lymphatics, a topic often overlooked, yet vital to the body's well-being. Among the attendees was Vanessa, a dietitian with a radiant presence, who was scheduled to speak about gut health. Little did I know our conversation would lead to a story of resilience, healing, and the incredible potential of the human body.

After my talk, Vanessa approached me, her curiosity piqued by the non-surgical methods I discussed. We exchanged pleasantries, and she eagerly inquired about my work, particularly my approach to eliminating scar tissue and restoring parts of the body that many medical professionals had written off as irreparable.

Vanessa's eyes gleamed with hope and skepticism as she shared her story. "Twelve months ago," she began, "I was in a severe motorbike accident in Spain. It was one of those moments that can change your life in an instant. I remember the sound of the crash, the pain that followed, and the overwhelming fear that my life would never be the same." Her voice trembled slightly, and I could see the emotional weight this memory still held for her.

The accident had shattered her left shoulder to bits. The doctors in Spain had given her the grim news: surgery was necessary to attempt to restore function to her arm. But Vanessa had a deep aversion to the idea of surgery. She knew that once the knife was taken to her body, there would be no going back, and she feared the unknown consequences.

So, she made a bold decision. "I didn't want surgery," she said firmly. "Instead, I sought other therapies. When I returned home to Bali, I immersed myself in the world of alternative healing. Bali is known for its incredible healers, and Vanessa was fortunate to work with some of the best. Physiotherapists, massage therapists—they all played a major role in realigning Vanessa's shoulder joint and increasing her range of movement."

Vanessa's journey was one of determination and perseverance. The therapies had helped, but they could only take her so far. Despite her progress, she still struggled with the simplest tasks— reaching behind her, stretching out her arm, and lifting light objects. "It was frustrating," Vanessa admitted. "I had come so far, yet I felt like I had hit a wall. The pain lingered, and the limitation in movement was a constant reminder of what I had lost."

As Vanessa spoke, I could see the desperation in her eyes, the yearning for a solution to finally bring her the relief she sought. I knew then that I could help her. "Vanessa," I said gently, "all we need to do is reduce the scar tissue around the head of your shoulder." The head of the shoulder refers to the area surrounding the rounded top portion of the shoulder joint, technically called the humeral head. This is the upper end of the humerus (upper arm bone) that fits into the glenoid cavity of the scapula (shoulder blade), forming the shoulder's ball-and-socket joint. "Once we do that, your body will realign itself, and healing will occur. The full range of movement will return. Also, we need to address the trauma in the tissues and the spine alignment."

Vanessa looked at me, her eyes wide with disbelief and hope. "Can it be that simple?" she asked.

I smiled. "The body is an incredible machine, Vanessa. It has an innate ability to heal itself, but sometimes it just needs a little guidance. Scar tissue can restrict movement and cause pain, but by carefully reducing it, we can allow the body to do what it is designed to do—heal."

As I explained the process to her, I saw hope return to her face. She had been through so much, yet here she was, ready to take another step toward reclaiming her life. I lived for this: helping people rediscover the power of their own bodies and showing them that healing was possible, even when it seemed out of reach.

Our meeting began a new chapter in Vanessa's healing journey. She left that day with a renewed sense of purpose, determined to give her body the chance to heal fully. Watching her walk away, I knew her story was far from over. It was a story of resilience, refusal to accept defeat, and the incredible things that can happen when we trust in the body's ability to heal itself.

Vanessa's transformation

Vanessa was set to leave for Bali in two weeks and was determined to transform her body to its best possible state before her departure. At 64, she carried the weight of emotional trauma and physical scars that had accumulated over a lifetime. The shattered shoulder from her motorbike accident in Spain was only part of the story. The more profound pain lay in the unhealed emotional wounds embedded in her tissues like anchors holding her back.

Recognizing the urgency of her situation, Vanessa booked eight sessions of non-surgical therapy and lymphatic drainage massage. During these sessions, I focused on key areas: her upper shoulders, lower spine, hips, her waistline, and around her stomach. These areas were not just physical focal points; they were the storage sites of her past traumas and unresolved emotions.

As I worked on her body, it became clear that Vanessa's issues were deeply rooted in her tissues. The body remembers what the mind tries to forget. These old wounds, stored in her subconscious, influenced how her physical self functioned. The scar tissues were more than just remnants of injuries—they were manifestations of the emotional pain she had carried for years.

Each session was a step toward releasing these burdens. As we worked through the layers of scar tissue, Vanessa felt physically and emotionally lighter. The non-surgical methods allowed us to renew and rejuvenate parts of her body that others deemed untreatable. Slowly but surely, her body responded, aligning with her renewed spirit.

We must remember that the issues in our tissues are often the main reasons we begin to fall apart. The body and mind are intricately connected, and unresolved emotions can manifest as physical pain and dysfunction. Vanessa's journey was a powerful reminder of this truth. By addressing both her physical and emotional scars, she was able to prepare not just for her trip to Bali but for a new chapter in her life, free from the weight of her past.

Vanessa couldn't believe it—her shoulder had regained its full range of motion, and her spine felt straighter than ever before. The alignment was perfect, a transformation she hadn't thought possible. But life, as it often does, threw her a curve ball.

While in Bali, Vanessa experienced a fall that left her hips aching and painful. Disheartened, she returned to her therapist in Bali for some relief and then dropped in to see me back in Melbourne for two more sessions. After those visits, she felt revitalized, her body strong and pain-free again.

With her newfound vitality, Vanessa was ready to conquer the world. As she prepared for a European trip, she couldn't help but think of her friend Chris. "Can you help him?" she asked, concerned. "He won't listen to me, and with his knees, I'm afraid he won't enjoy our trip."

For a week, Vanessa talked to Chris about me, trying to convince him to see me. Reluctantly, Chris finally agreed, although he was skeptical. He thought the treatment would never work and that traveling to Melbourne was too much hassle. Vanessa knew Chris would be just as amazed by the results, and they would be ready to embark on their adventure together without anything holding them back.

35   CATHY

The belly button mystery

Cathy had always been intrigued by the body's hidden networks, especially the lymphatic system. When she learned that a new lymphatic specialist had joined the clinic in Blackburn, just before the world changed with the pandemic, she booked a session out of curiosity and a desire for relief.

The clinic was a sanctuary of peace, and Cathy immediately felt drawn to the SOQI bed—a marvel of holistic healing. Its gentle waves of energy and the soothing touch of a lymphatic massage made the hour-long session feel like a journey into serenity. But beneath Cathy's calm exterior was a troubling discomfort that she could no longer ignore.

As we worked together, Cathy began to open up about the pain haunting her. It lingered around her waistline, a constant companion that left her bloated and sore. Cathy couldn't pinpoint its origin, and no matter how hard she tried, the weight clung stubbornly to her frame, adding to her misery. Her legs were perpetually aching, and every day felt like a battle against an invisible enemy.

During the session, I focused on her waistline, particularly around her belly button. I sensed that something was amiss but was unsure what it could be. The session ended with Cathy feeling lighter and more at ease, but what happened later that night left us astounded.

As Cathy was getting ready for bed, she felt an odd sensation at her belly button. To her utter horror, a cotton tip emerged from it. Her mind raced, trying to comprehend what was happening. The words escaped her in a panicked whisper, "What the hell is going on?"

Then, Cathy remembered a seemingly innocent habit she'd had for as long as she could recall—cleaning her belly button with cotton tips. It dawned on her that over the years, some of those tips must have broken off and become lodged inside, unbeknownst to her. The realization hit hard, especially when she acknowledged that what she had dismissed as a mild, persistent odor was now a full-blown stench.

Cathy's discovery was as shocking as it was eye-opening. It underscored the hidden complexities of the human body and the way seemingly minor habits can lead to significant consequences. At that moment, Cathy knew she had found more than just a practitioner—she had found a path to understanding her body's signals, no matter how unexpected.

Cathy returned for many more sessions, determined to clear the waste from her body. Over time, her body responded, and she began to feel amazing. To her surprise, more cotton tips emerged from her belly button, a bizarre but telling sign of our deep work.

Just before Easter, Cathy experienced intense pain. She couldn't figure out what was wrong and due to the holiday closures, could not reach her regular doctor. Desperate, she tried the local hospital, but that didn't yield any results either. Eventually, Cathy managed to see a specialist who suggested an ultrasound to check for a possible hernia. But with everything closed down for the Easter break, she was left in excruciating pain, forced to rely on painkillers as she headed home.

The next day, Cathy came to see me. I suggested a gentle lymphatic massage, hoping it might bring some relief. It wasn't much of a solution, but it was all I could offer. As the day passed, the pain gradually subsided, and Cathy finally found some relief.

Had the doctors seen her, Cathy would have undoubtedly gone down the path of surgery, which might have been a valid option. But this approach spared Cathy from unnecessary pain, recovery time, and significant expenses.

Five years later, Cathy remains a regular client, a testament to the power of the body's ability to heal when given the proper support. Her journey reminds us that the most straightforward solutions sometimes save us from challenging problems.

36   BRIAN AND KERRY

Why do we wait?

It was New Year's Eve 2023, and I wasn't particularly excited about going out. The last few years had kept many of us indoors, celebrating the turn of the year in quieter ways, thanks to the pandemic. But this year, I decided to step out to mark the occasion with a night of music at a local RSL club. The crowd was mostly over sixty—people looking to reminisce and enjoy a bit of dancing as they welcomed what we all hoped would be a fantastic year.

At our table, I met Kerry and Brian, part of a lively group of ten. The conversation quickly turned to health—a topic that naturally comes up when I'm surrounded by people in their sixties and beyond. We discussed the usual diet, exercise, and the importance of regular check-ups. We all knew what we should be doing, yet so many of us waited until the last minute—until that dreaded test result from the doctor forced us to confront the reality we'd been avoiding.

It's a strange thing. We know what to do, but we don't do it. We ignore the signs, pushing them aside until they're too loud to dismiss. Sitting there, listening to Kerry and Brian share their own stories of close calls and wake-up calls, I couldn't help but think about how common this was. The fear of the unknown, the terror of a diagnosis that might drop us to the ground, keeps us paralyzed. We wait until we're faced with something profound, something we can no longer ignore, before we take action.

Why do we wait until it's almost too late?

As the clock struck midnight, the room erupted in cheers, and confetti filled the air, welcoming 2024 with a bang. Three of the couples at the table had battled cancer. They were still grappling with the aftermath of their treatments, the lingering effects of dangerous drugs casting a shadow over their lives. The conversation turned back to health, and Brian, with a mixture of bravado and disbelief, remarked, "That will never happen to me."

Brian and his wife, Kerry, were particularly intrigued by my profession. Kerry, a self-proclaimed health nut, had survived breast cancer years ago. Determined to keep cancer at bay, she had opted for surgery but refused drugs. On the other hand, Brian was a high-stress individual, balancing the demands of work and life. Despite the challenges, they both seemed to enjoy life, though the strain was evident in Brian's demeanor.

As the night wore on, we shared stories, laughter, and hope for the future. We said our goodbyes, and I watched as the new year began, unaware of the journey that awaited them.

Fast forward to April, and Kerry and Brian walked into my clinic, their faces etched with worry. "Hi, how are you both doing?" I asked, sensing the weight of their visit.

Kerry's voice trembled as she began to speak, "Oh Michelle, Brian has just finished eight rounds of radiation for throat cancer, and he's a mess. He can't eat, has no energy, is losing weight, and it's like he has no life left in him."

As Kerry spoke, I saw the toll the last few months had taken on Brian. He had aged considerably, his once vibrant energy replaced by a tired and weary expression. The stress and fear were palpable.

A year ago, they had booked an overseas trip, a dream vacation with their family. But now, with the trip only four weeks away, Brian was adamant that he couldn't go. "There's no way I can walk far, let alone enjoy a trip overseas," he said, his voice laced with defeat.

Kerry's eyes pleaded with me, seeking a glimmer of hope that Brian would find the strength to make the journey. This pivotal moment would test their resilience and the healing power of the body and mind. The path ahead was uncertain, but as I listened to their story, I knew this unexpected journey was just beginning.

A turnaround worth millions

Kerry and Brian had been through more than their fair share of challenges. With Brian's ongoing battle with throat cancer and Kerry's persistent back pain and tennis elbow, their future seemed uncertain. They both agreed when I suggested we try two sessions a week of non-surgical therapies combined with lymphatic drainage massage. Kerry was eager to find relief, and though Brian was skeptical, he admitted he had nothing to lose. "I'll teach you how to heal yourself," I said, laughing, knowing this was just the beginning of their journey.

From the very first session, both noticed a difference. Brian, weighed down by doubt, began to feel a glimmer of hope. Kerry, with her chronic pain and kyphosis—an increased curve of the upper back, likely due to the aftereffects of her breast cancer—felt her posture improving as the tension in her shoulders eased. The non-surgical treatments and a heart-release technique worked wonders for her.

After just three weeks, the transformation was undeniable. Kerry mentioned how Brian was now excited about their upcoming European trip, a holiday they had feared would be impossible. His energy was returning, and even though his throat was still tender, his specialist had reassured him that full recovery could take up to a year.

They left for their dream holiday, and when they returned five weeks later, the change in both was remarkable. They were glowing with health and happiness. Brian's energy was better than it had been in years, and Kerry's back pain was a distant memory. They continued to see me every two weeks to maintain the regeneration of their cells, and during one of those sessions, they shared some incredible news.

Brian had gone to his doctor to receive an update on his cancer diagnosis. They were emotional when they walked into my clinic later that afternoon. Tears filled their eyes as they told me, "The cancer is gone... it no longer exists."

37   CHRIS

A journey of transformation

"Wow!" Vanessa couldn't contain her excitement. "That's so, so good! I'm going to forward this to my girlfriend for her husband!" She was talking about Chris, her partner, who had finally taken the step she had hoped for.

Vanessa had been seeing me for two weeks and shared her concern during one of our sessions. "I wish Chris would come and see you. His knees are killing him, and we're heading off to Europe in a few months. I'm worried he won't be able to enjoy the trip. Walking will be a real effort for him."

I understood her frustration. "Vanessa," I said, "I often hear this call to action, but the first step to healing is wanting to get well. You can't force anyone to heal themselves."

Vanessa nodded in agreement. "It's so frustrating, but you're right. He has to want it."

Then, to my surprise and delight, Chris booked an appointment. Fantastic! At 67 years old, Chris was grappling with multiple health issues. Like a fluid ball, a swollen elbow was one of the most noticeable. I immediately suggested, "You should get that drained."

"That's great, Michelle," Chris replied. "I'm actually booked in to see my doctor tomorrow to have it drained."

Chris had been an avid cyclist for decades, maintaining a fitness level. However, he didn't realize that his body was suffering from severe dehydration. Despite not feeling thirsty, his ligaments and tendons were incredibly tight, stiff, and inflexible. Every time he worked out, his body was under enormous stress.

I knew we had work to do. Hydration was the first critical step in Chris's healing journey. I explained to him the importance of water in maintaining physical fitness and overall health. His body needed replenishment and rejuvenation to restore flexibility and ease his pain.

As we began his sessions, I could see the difference it was making. Slowly but surely, Chris's body responded. Once a source of constant pain, his knees began to feel more flexible. His elbow, once drained, healed remarkably well. The tightness in his ligaments and tendons eased as his body became better hydrated.

Vanessa was overjoyed. Chris's transformation meant that their upcoming trip to Europe, which had seemed daunting, was something they could both look forward to with excitement. The miracle of healing wasn't just in the physical changes but in Chris's newfound belief in his body's ability to recover and thrive. Also, his once over-size waste was slowly reducing; another bonus of lymphatic drainage massage and non-surgical health.

This journey was not just about alleviating pain; it was about restoring hope, renewing the spirit, and realizing the potential within every person to heal and flourish, no matter their age or condition. As Chris and Vanessa prepared for their adventure abroad, I knew they were embarking on more than just a vacation—they were stepping into a new chapter of their lives: health, happiness, and possibility.

38   MICHAEL AND SIBILA

In 2024, I embarked on a mission to become the best teacher I could be, fuelled by an insatiable desire to share the incredible knowledge I had accumulated. My goal was to revolutionize the healing world through the art of Lymphology and lymphatic massage. This journey began with a series of educational workshops open to anyone eager to learn how to heal themselves and their loved ones, or even pursue a rewarding career in health.

In January 2024, I hosted my first weekend workshop, a pivotal moment that would set the stage for something truly extraordinary.

Six incredible individuals gathered to learn from me, and though I was initially nervous, I quickly found my stride. My natural teaching abilities emerged, and the energy in the room became electric.

One of the attendees was Sibila, a school librarian from Sydney, New South Wales. She had previously attended a non-surgical course with me in Coffs Harbour and had experienced the profound effects of a lymphatic drainage session. That experience ignited a spark within her—a desire for a more meaningful purpose in life, leading her to pursue a career in health.

Sibila brought her partner, Michael, along for the weekend. While she delved into the course, Michael explored Melbourne. However, on the second day, an emergency caused one participant to leave, creating an uneven number of our partner exercises in lymphatic massage. Sibila invited Michael to join us, and he graciously accepted.

Michael, a former ambulance driver whose career had been upended by the Covid-19 pandemic, brought to the group a wealth of medical knowledge. His input was invaluable, and his presence was warmly welcomed.

During the afternoon session, Michael asked if I could work on his back, as he had been suffering from chronic pain that had made sleep nearly impossible. I placed him on the SOQI bed for 30 minutes, followed by 30 minutes of non-surgical treatment on the massage table. I focused on his middle to upper back and then moved to the lower back, guiding him to relax and breathe deeply.

I asked for guidance as I worked, knowing I intended to bring healing. Michael rose from the table with a look of wonder—he couldn't quite describe how he felt, but something had undeniably shifted. That night, for the first time in what seemed like an eternity, Michael slept peacefully, free from pain.

The transformation was nothing short of miraculous. Michael's body had shifted from a state of stress and survival to one of healing and renewal. Michael was amazed at how something so gentle could create such profound change. This experience was a testament to the incredible power of Lymphology—a power that I am determined to share with the world.

This record is just the beginning. My workshops are not merely educational; they are life-changing experiences. Anyone willing to learn has the potential to heal, transform, and live a life of purpose. My journey as a teacher has only just begun, but the impact is already rippling outwards, creating a wave of healing that will continue to grow. The best-seller I'm writing is more than a book—it's a movement worth a million that will change lives forever.

39   ROSS

Ross had been a loyal client of Chris, his trusted hairdresser, for over three decades. Their relationship extended beyond mere haircuts; it was a bond formed through shared stories, life's ups and downs, and a mutual respect that had grown over the years. One day, while sitting in Chris's chair, Ross revealed a harrowing chapter of his life—a battle with cancer that had taken a toll on his body and spirit. The cancer had manifested as a tumor beneath his left eye, leading to surgery that left him with a metal plate inserted above his jawline. The surgery saved his life, but it also left him with a swollen eye, blurred vision, and a constant reminder of his fragility.

Ross's ordeal didn't end with the surgery. The relentless pandemic had thrown the world into chaos, and Ross was caught in the whirlwind. Due to the overwhelming strain on the healthcare system, his follow-up with the surgeon was delayed indefinitely. Stuck in limbo, Ross was prescribed continuous antibiotics, the only measure to keep potential infections at bay. But these antibiotics came with their challenges, ravaging his body's good bacteria and leaving his immune system struggling to cope.

Chris, who had always been more than just a hairdresser to Ross, listened intently to his story. He knew someone who might be able to help—a Lymphology practitioner named Michelle, who had an incredible reputation for her work in healing the body through non-invasive therapies. Chris shared Michelle's profession with Ross, planting a seed of hope in his mind. Ross, who remembered his father speaking of lymphatic drainage almost 80 years ago, felt a spark of curiosity. He was desperate for relief and was willing to explore any avenue that could offer him some respite from the pain and discomfort.

The following week, Ross decided to give it a try. He began sessions with me, starting with the SOQI bed and lymphatic drainage around his face. The journey wasn't easy; it required patience, commitment, and an open mind. But slowly, week by week, Ross began to notice a change. The swelling around his eye started diminishing, his vision gradually improved, and the pain became more bearable. After about eight weeks of regular sessions, Ross's eye maintained a reasonable level of vision, and the swelling significantly reduced. I told Ross the antibiotics killed the harmful and good bacteria, weakening his immune system. However, Ross, a man of resolve, trusted his doctors and continued with the antibiotics for another two and a half years.

Finally, the day came when Ross was able to see his surgeon. The metal plate that had been a constant reminder of his battle was removed, and with it, a new chapter of healing began. Ross continued his sessions with me, allowing his body to heal naturally, free from the burden of foreign materials and harsh medications. His eye, once a source of pain and distress, now looked fantastic. His vision, which the trauma of surgery and illness had clouded, was now one hundred percent better.

But the most remarkable transformation was in Ross's spirit. He had always been a man who faced life head-on, but now, with his health restored, he found a new zest for living. He threw himself into his hobbies and work with renewed energy, understanding that true wealth was not in material possessions but in the health and vitality that allowed him to live fully. Ross's positive outlook, combined with my expertise, had set him on a journey of recovery and thriving. He still pops in now and then to say hello, a reminder of the incredible power of resilience, hope, and the right kind of healing.

40 JENNY

Jenny made an appointment and came to my clinic in early 2023, burdened by years of stress and inflammation that left her knees on the brink of exploding with pain. A beautiful woman in her late sixties, Jenny had struggled to lose weight and found herself at a loss when the doctors offered no solutions beyond pain medication and other drugs she was already on. Determined to avoid this path, Jenny sought a different way forward.

During our first session, Jenny's knees and back felt noticeably better. I then gave her a few simple tasks at home, such as focusing on deep breathing and becoming more aware of her stress. During this discussion, Jenny came to a critical realization.

For forty years, she had lived with a husband she felt little connection with except for companionship. Her older son, still living at home, showed little respect for her, and her grandchildren added to the chaos under her roof. The weight of these strained relationships and unrelenting responsibilities had taken a toll on her heart, manifesting as chronic inflammation and pain throughout her body. The root of Jenny's physical distress was apparent stress was the true culprit behind her chronic pain, and recognizing this was the first step towards her healing journey.

Jenny's journey with us was one of quiet courage and constant battle. She longed to come every week, finding solace and clarity in the sessions that helped her understand her pain and gain a sharper focus on her life. Yet, as someone not the primary breadwinner, Jenny found it difficult to ask for money to invest in her health, even though she knew how much it was helping her. She often brought home-cooked sweets to the clinic, a gesture of gratitude and a sign of a more profound struggle. Jenny was an emotional eater, and sugar had become her constant companion, a comfort amid her turmoil. She knew it wasn't good for her, yet it was the only way she could feel something, even if that feeling was fleeting and ultimately unsatisfying.

It was heartbreaking to witness Jenny's inner conflict, her desire for change overshadowed by a lack of strength to break free. Over six months, as she continued her sessions, Jenny experienced moments of triumph. She felt great after swimming at the gym, and there was a period when she cut down on her sugar intake. Then winter came, and with it, the swimming stopped, and the cycle of life's crises began to spin again.

Despite her progress, Jenny never fully permitted herself to heal. Deep down, she knew that if she grew stronger, she would have to confront the reality of her marriage—a relationship that had long since ceased to bring her joy or fulfillment. The fear of leaving, of stepping into the unknown without a clear path forward, kept her from embracing the change she so desperately needed.

Jenny's story poignantly reminds us of the complexities of healing. It's not just about the physical pain or symptoms we can see; it's about the emotional and psychological barriers that hold us back. For Jenny, healing meant facing the truth about her life, and that was a step she wasn't ready to take. So, Jenny remained in the cycle, her heart heavy with the knowledge of what could be, but her feet rooted in the familiar ground of what was.

41   MANDY

In 2016, I stood at the precipice of a new chapter, freshly minted as a life coach, after working as a personal trainer for 15 years. The thrill of helping others reclaim their health was an ever-present fire in my heart, but I was still finding my footing, eager yet uncertain of where this journey would lead. Little did I know that the arrival of one woman at my small health retreat would shape my career and deepen my understanding of the true essence of healing.

Our retreat, in an elusive suburb of Melbourne, offered a week-long, all-inclusive live-in program. It was a sanctuary designed to nurture the body and soul, where our guests could disconnect from the chaos of life and reconnect with themselves. The program was my labor of love, crafted with care to address the unique needs of each person who crossed our threshold. And that's where Mandy came in—a woman whose strength and resolve left an indelible mark on my soul and still has stayed connected.

Mandy had traveled down from the coast of New South Wales, seeking more than just a respite from her daily life. Mandy was dealing with breast cancer, a diagnosis that had shaken her world to its core. But Mandy was not one to surrender, determined to explore every avenue to restore her health and well-being. She had heard whispers about people's transformative experiences at our retreat, stories of dissolving health issues that seemed insurmountable. So, with hope and trepidation, she walked through our doors.

From the moment we met, I knew Mandy was different. She had a quiet strength and resilience that belied the seriousness of her condition. She was ready to win, but not in the conventional sense. Mandy sought to heal from within, to empower her body to fight the disease on its terms with as little interference from Western medicine as possible. It was a bold decision, one that resonated deeply with me.

We spent the week together, delving into the intricacies of nutrition and its impact on the immune system. Amanda, our resident nutritionist, was integral to Mandy's journey. Her expertise in low-inflammation foods was crucial in designing a diet that supported Mandy's immune system while helping her body eliminate waste effectively. Every meal was a carefully curated experience designed to nourish Mandy's body and, more importantly, her spirit.

Mandy's transformation was nothing short of miraculous. By the end of the week, she had shed three dress sizes and looked a decade younger. Her skin glowed with vitality, and there was a light in her eyes that hadn't been there when she first arrived. But it wasn't just her physical appearance that had changed. There was a newfound confidence in Mandy, a belief that she could overcome anything life threw her way.

After the retreat, Mandy did chemo treatment, but she made a bold decision to continue her healing journey with minimal reliance on Western medicine. She wanted to take control of her health, to be the master of her destiny. And in doing so, she taught me an invaluable lesson: true healing is as much about the mind and spirit as it is about the body.

A battle beyond the surface

Mandy left my health retreat on a high, brimming with newfound energy and determination. She had dropped three dress sizes, looked ten years younger, and had a clear vision of how she wanted to continue her journey. But beneath the surface, Mandy's life was far from healed.

Returning home, Mandy was immediately thrust back into the chaos of her reality. Her husband's ongoing issues with a stroke weighed heavily on her, filling her with constant concern and fear. They were also grappling with the decision to sell their 24/7 holiday park business, which had drained them physically and emotionally. Mandy longed to return to their peaceful mountain getaway, where she could breathe freely again. But there were deeper wounds that had yet to heal, wounds that no amount of fresh air could mend.

Mandy's struggles were rooted in more than just her present circumstances. She carried with her the pain of a lifetime, particularly the unresolved issues of abandonment from her mother. These emotional scars manifested in her body as stored waste, particularly in her breasts. If not addressed, this waste doesn't simply disappear—it festers. Over time, it can become lumpy, infected, and ridden with microorganisms that slowly begin to rot the body from within. We call this process cancer.

As a Lymphologist, I've learned that breasts, once they've fulfilled their role of nourishing life, often become storage grounds for emotional and physical waste. It's a harsh reality that all women face, whether they admit it or not. I don't care what anyone says—all women have lumpy breasts, even myself. The challenge lies in understanding how to deal with the emotional trauma trapped in breast tissue.

Mandy's journey was not just about shedding pounds or looking younger—it was about confronting the deep-seated emotions that had taken root in her body. The fear, the pain, the unresolved anger—they all needed to be released. And that's where the real work began. Over the next couple of years, we stayed in contact; Mandy was also searching to find another way to try and get rid of the lump. It seemed, at times, it grew, and at other times it shrank. It seemed it would change from soft to hard often.

In 2023, Mandy took a bold step toward reclaiming her health and vitality by coming to Melbourne for a remarkable 16-day water fast. It was an awe-inspiring journey of determination and resilience that left Mandy feeling rejuvenated and more alive than ever. The day after she completed her fast, I worked on a persistent lump using non-surgical techniques, and the results were nothing short of miraculous. Mandy was so impressed with the SOQI bed that she purchased one for her country retreat.

Mandy's retreat, nestled in the serene countryside, is now thriving—where others find the same healing and renewal she experienced. It's a sanctuary of wellness and transformation, and I'm proud to say it's featured at the back of this book as a recommended destination for those seeking proper health.

After a decade of hard work, Mandy and her husband finally sold their holiday park, which brought them much joy and relief. Now, they can entirely focus on their health retreat and embrace life.

Mandy, your journey has been nothing short of extraordinary. Love you, Mandy.

Mandy's story is about courage, determination, and the power of self-belief. It was the beginning of my realization that healing is a deeply personal journey that requires more than just physical intervention. It requires a shift in mindset, a belief in the body's innate ability to heal, and the courage to take the road less traveled. For me, it was the beginning of a lifelong mission to guide others on their healing journeys, one step at a time.

42   PAUL

In 2024, Paul, a determined man in his early fifties, stumbled across my name while searching desperately for a solution to the relentless pain in his hips. For years, the pain had taken over his life, stealing his joy and making every step an agonizing reminder that something was wrong. Doctors had repeatedly suggested hip surgery, a standard but invasive procedure that Paul instinctively knew wasn't the answer for him. He believed there had to be another way, a method not just to mask the pain but to truly heal his body.

Paul's intuition led him to my practice, where he tried my methods. From the moment he walked through the door, I could see the weariness in his eyes—the kind that comes from enduring chronic pain and endless medical appointments. But there was also a spark of hope, a belief that he was on the verge of something transformative.

Paul's case was straightforward, yet profound. His body was dehydrated, and his spine was out of alignment, causing the hips to bear the brunt of the discomfort. It wasn't a matter of complex surgeries or medications; it was about realigning his body and rehydrating the tissues that had become brittle and inflamed over time.

For the next five weeks, Paul committed to his healing journey, visiting me once a week. Each session began with thirty minutes in the SOQI bed, a therapeutic device that helped his body relax and prepare for the more profound work. I then focused on lymphatic drainage, carefully working to clear the crystallizations that had formed around his spine and hip area. These crystallizations, often ignored by conventional medicine, were the culprits behind his pain, restricting movement and causing inflammation.

With each session, Paul felt the pain in his hips receding, replaced by a sense of ease and fluidity he hadn't experienced in years. By the end of the fifth week, the pain that had once dominated his life was gone. Paul's body had responded beautifully to the treatments, realigning itself and restoring the natural flow of energy that had been blocked for so long.

Paul's story didn't end there. Though his hips no longer ached, he visited me occasionally for health checks and chats, ensuring his body remained in optimal condition. His journey was a testament to the power of the body's innate ability to heal when given the proper support. In just five weeks, Paul had not only avoided surgery but had reclaimed his life, proving that true healing comes from understanding and working with the body, not against it.

Paul's story became a beacon of hope for many others, a shining example of what was possible when one trusted in the body's ability to heal. The simplicity of his treatment contrasted starkly with the complex solutions often proposed by modern medicine, reinforcing the idea that sometimes, the best solutions are the most natural ones.

43   MICHELLE

In 2018, a client who had traveled to Mexico for a unique experience told me about Darrell Wolfe, whose approach to health was unlike anything I'd encountered before. They urged me to connect with him, mentioning that Darrell would be coming to Australia in 2023. The timing seemed perfect, and I knew this was an opportunity I couldn't miss.

I immersed myself in Darrell's teachings for two months, attending his "Life" and highly regarded "non-surgical" courses. I was instantly captivated when I watched Darrell live for the first time. His unfiltered truth and bold approach to health resonated deeply with me, especially given my background as a Lymphologist. Everything he said connected with what I knew, but with an added layer of depth and understanding.

I contacted Darrell and organized an event near my clinic. The turnout was incredible—over 90 people from across Melbourne came together, eager to learn. The success of that event led to another, an all-day workshop the following Monday, where the energy and enthusiasm were even higher.

At the time, lymphology was already producing excellent results, but I couldn't help but wonder—what if I combined it with

Darrell's non-surgical methods? Non-surgical work is, without a doubt, the most potent bodywork on the planet, and I have over 100 case studies to prove it.

My journey with Darrell's techniques was nothing short of remarkable. Over six weeks, I learned the intricate art of non-surgical healing, delving into the power of removing crystallization, calcification, and inflammation—issues that plague the body and drown the very essence of life. What began as a personal exploration quickly became a transformative experience for everyone around me.

This chapter in my life wasn't just about acquiring new skills but expanding the boundaries of what's possible in healing. My work with Lymphology was powerful, but it became unstoppable with the addition of non-surgical techniques. The results were undeniable, and the impact on my clients was profound.

This journey of discovery and healing isn't just a chapter in my life; it's a cornerstone of this book that will inspire millions, offering hope and real solutions to those seeking proper health.

44   DI

The burden of silence

Before the world changed in 2019, I met a woman named Di. She was one of my earliest clients from Blackburn. Di was in her sixties, a naturopath who began her journey in the early 1960s. She carried with her a lifetime of knowledge but also a lifetime of pain.

Di's body had become a battlefield. Multiple conditions burdened her. Her weight had spiraled out of control, and she had undergone surgeries for her bladder, gallbladder, and the veins that bulge angrily from her legs. These physical ailments were the visible scars of a deeper, hidden wound.

Di was once a radiant beauty, a model in the vibrant and wild seventies. But beneath the surface, she harbored a secret that had haunted her since she was a teenager. Di had been raped, a violent act that shattered her sense of self and left her with emotional scars that would fester for decades. She buried this trauma deep within, locking it away where no-one could see. But the weight of that secret, the burden of silence, grew heavier each year.

As the years went by, Di's body became a fortress, a layer of protection against a world that had hurt her so deeply. The weight piled on, serving as armor to keep her safe from the memories she couldn't bear to confront. But as her body expanded, so did her self-loathing. She despised the reflection in the mirror, seeing only the physical manifestation of her pain. The hatred for her body was like wildfire, consuming her from the inside out and fueling even more health issues, particularly in her gut, the very core of her being.

Despite her expertise as a naturopath and an emotional healer, Di found herself powerless to heal the most important person in her life—herself. She knew the principles of health and understood the intricate workings of the human body, but she was lost when it came to her own. The weight of her past, the trauma she had never spoken of, was a chain that kept her bound in a prison of her own making.

In Di, I saw the embodiment of so many women who have walked through life carrying the weight of unspeakable experiences, their pain hidden behind brave faces. Di's story was not unique, but it was devastatingly real. The secret she had kept for so long had become the very thing that was destroying her. And at that moment, I knew that her healing journey would not just be about shedding physical weight but about confronting the emotional weight that had been crushing her spirit for decades.

Finding home amid the chaos

Di loved coming to see me—not just for the soothing comfort of the lymphatic drainage massages but also for the warmth of our conversations. The world had turned upside down, and like many, she found solace in the company of a stranger. Her home life was a different story. After thirty years of marriage, she and her husband were locked in a silent battle, their relationship strained by the divisive issues surrounding Covid-19. Di was adamant in her beliefs, vehemently opposed to anything the government suggested, and this clash of opinions had driven a wedge between them.

Di made an unusual offer one day after a session: "Would you like some cats?" It wasn't the first time we'd talked about animals. Di was an animal lover, and our affection for creatures often entered our chats. Although I had always loved animals, my lifestyle wasn't ideal for a dog, and I had never seriously considered adopting a cat. But something about the way Di asked made me listen closely.

Di explained that her son's best friends, a couple living in a small apartment, were desperate to find a new home for their two cats. Yoski, a young alley cat, and Hatrick, a six-year-old ginger, had grown up together. The couple, who I'll call Sue and her girlfriend, had faced unimaginable challenges during the pandemic. They were a gay couple, both hesitant about the Covid-19 vaccine, but the pressures of maintaining a livelihood in those uncertain times forced their hand.

Sue ultimately decided to get the vaccine, but what followed was tragic. She suffered a sudden cardiac arrest and was rushed to the hospital, where she narrowly survived. The experience left Sue and her partner devastated, but they had no choice but to continue, hoping for the best as life progressed.

However, their fears were compounded when it came time for the second dose. Despite reassurances from doctors, Sue once again faced severe complications—this time, she didn't survive. Within 24 hours, she passed away, leaving her partner in unbearable grief. The heartbreak didn't end there. Sue's partner, who had been unable to accompany Sue to the hospital due to her unvaccinated status, was consumed by despair. Two weeks later, she took her own life, unable to bear the weight of her loss.

The couple's beloved cats were left behind, now homeless and in need of care. Sue's mother took them in, but the emotional toll of losing her daughter and the overwhelming grief that followed was almost too much to bear. Meeting her and seeing the pain etched into her face, I felt the full impact of the tragedy. These were not just stories in the news; they were real people, lives torn apart by circumstances no-one could have predicted.

When I visited Sue's mother to meet the cats, the emotional rollercoaster of the pandemic hit me anew. The anguish in that home was palpable, a stark reminder of the lives lost and the loved ones left behind. But amid that sorrow, Yoski and Hatrick were a beacon of hope, looking for a new beginning—a home where they could be safe and loved again.

A journey of healing and light

As we arrived at our country estate, with its vast 10 acres of open space, it was as if Yoski and Hatrick had found a slice of heaven amid the hellish times we had all endured. It took nearly two months for these two once-frightened cats to muster the courage to explore their new surroundings, slowly emerging from their hiding places under chairs and in dark corners. But when they did, it was beautiful to witness their transformation—blossoming from a place of fear into one of love and light.

Now, three years later, Yoski and Hatrick are never home. They constantly roam the land, reveling in their newfound freedom. They walk with us whenever we are outside, basking in the sunshine and fresh air, their joy infectious and their spirits unbreakable. I keep in touch with Sue's mother, sharing photos of the cats and the life we've built together on this peaceful estate. It's a reminder that life is indeed a journey, not a destination.

Little did I know these two cats would become so much more than just pets. They became a source of comfort, healing, and connection during one of the most challenging periods in recent history. As the world struggled to recover from the pandemic's grip, Yoski and Hatrick stood as symbols of resilience and the enduring power of love, even amidst overwhelming loss. Their journey mirrored our own—a testament to the strength of love and the light that can emerge from even the darkest places.

45   JUTTA

A global healing revolution

I met Jutta in Coffs Harbour in 2023 while doing the non–surgical course run by Darrell Wolfe. Although I didn't connect with her very much, she is still a beautiful lady who wants to change how we see healthcare. When she returned home, she had made up her mind to open her retreat.

Jutta's retreat quickly became a beacon of hope and healing in Victoria. Her wisdom, combined with the advanced techniques she learned, attracted people from all walks of life. The retreat was more than just a place for physical recovery; it became a center for holistic healing, nurturing the mind, body, and spirit.

Together, we envisioned a world where Lymphology Australia would set the standard for healthcare, revolutionizing how people approach illness and wellness. Jutta's retreat was the first step in a grander plan to establish healing centers worldwide, each dedicated to the principles of Lymphology and non-surgical recovery.

Jutta's journey from a motel owner to a leader in global health is a testament to the power of vision and determination. Her story is an inspiration, and her retreat models what's possible when passion meets purpose. Her work is a vital part of the global revolution in healthcare, and Lymphology Australia is leading the charge.

Jutta's own words 2024

> *I reached a fork in the road when my world changed forever on New Year's Eve 1994. When I got the call that my mother had died suddenly in her sleep in Las Vegas while visiting her sisters— a family reunion after not seeing each other for over 30 years!!*
>
> *Long story short—the journey of dealing with my mother's sudden death—made me vow that I'd never trust the medical system ever again. I started my new journey of awakenings on how we all have been lied to about many things, especially about our bodies and how they can heal themselves if they are given all the conditions needed to be able to self-heal. We are our healers, and Mother Nature and her offerings enable the body to reconnect with itself and heal.*

I researched, learned, and participated in many modalities. Still, I came across Darrell Wolfe in 2020, doing one of his "one a day" and it had me spellbound with the truths he was speaking. It all resonated with me, every word. I continued researching. Darrell had an extensive library to investigate. It made such sense, and most of it is common sense. Plus, there were lots of links for peer-reviewed research.

Then it happened—Darrell announced that he was coming to Australia!! I had to be there, by hook or by crook, to take advantage of this window of opportunity.

It was a life-changing experience, and I'm forever blessed that I was able to participate in the three certifications that Darrell offered. The ability to look at things differently and let go of things that no longer served any purpose enabled me to move forward with love and joy in my heart for myself and everyone else in and around my life. I started to get excited about my future, as I was retired at this stage. My husband and I sold the motel, our business for the last 17 years of my life, just before the pandemic hit. I had less time in front of me—in the future— than what I had behind me, and I was slowly fading. Still, after doing the Whole Life Coach, Wolfe Non-Surgical, and the sacred feminine certification, I'm excited about all possibilities! My ability to teach others and enable them to heal themselves with the wisdom and knowledge I shared triggered visions and faith that humanity will do better once they know better. Little by little, one person at a time.

During the course, I met Michelle Richardson, and unknowingly then, I had no idea what impact she would have on my life in the future. Minding my own business, it came to my attention that a few members doing the course with me were having Michelle give them lymphatic drainage in the evenings. I still didn't think much about it and its importance. Then, much later, other members traveled to Melbourne. They did Michelle's lymphatic drainage training at her clinic in Belgrave. This piqued my interest, and I started to follow Michelle on Facebook. From then on, I decided that I had to find out more information for myself, so I then did the certification in lymphatic drainage with Michelle. I was impressed with Michelle's training and wanted more, so I'm doing further certification with Karl West of the International Academy of Lymphology to become a certified Lymphologist. I am close to completing my certification, but I will continue to further my knowledge, wisdom, and understanding through time and distance of how this amazing body we have all been gifted works, and how we can heal ourselves physically, mentally, spiritually, and emotionally.

It's my passion and purpose to show others how to help themselves if they are willing to do the work.

46   TRACEY

A journey back

I was born in Rhodesia, which is now Zimbabwe. My family moved to South Africa when I was seven because of the civil war in Zimbabwe. The closest big town to where I currently live is Queenstown. I was cancer-free for many years before coming to study with Darrell and to be trained to open my clinic in South

Africa. My brother immigrated to Australia in 2012, and my mother immigrated in 2005. They were both in SA until then.

In August 2023, I met Tracey during a Non-Surgical certification course in the tranquil setting of New South Wales. We formed an immediate bond, and there was an undeniable connection as if our paths had been destined to cross. Tracey bore a large scar stretching from her neck to her chin, a constant reminder of the battle she had fought. The scar was not just physical; the swelling that accompanied it was a manifestation of the unresolved trauma her body had endured.

Tracey's journey to healing had led her to Darrell Wolfe, a man she deeply admired for his incredible knowledge and expertise in regenerating the body. He had become her mentor, guiding her through the complex landscape of holistic health. Her respect for Darrell was palpable, and she spoke of him with a reverence reserved for those who have profoundly touched her life.

As we worked together, I could see the determination in Tracey's eyes. She was a woman on a mission to heal her body and reclaim her life. Our connection grew stronger with each session, and I felt privileged to be a part of her journey.

The work had to be done

In our group session, Darrell invited anyone open to it to let him work on them. Tracey, hesitant but determined, raised her hand. She was visibly anxious, her body tensing as she lay on the floor allowing Darrell better access to her neck.

Using his elbow, Darrell began working deep into the sensitive area, and I could see Tracey's unease turn into panic. This was not just a physical pain she was confronting; it was something far more pro-found. For Tracey, those few minutes felt like an eternity. I watched closely, witnessing what seemed like an out-of-body experience as Darrell guided her through the process. His presence was grounding, pulling her back into the moment as he continued his work.

When he finished, Darrell instructed Tracey to rest and relax. The energy in the room was palpable—three words echoed in my mind: Wow, Wow, Wow. The next day, I asked Tracey how she was feeling. Her response was thoughtful. "Do you think the tumour will come back?" she asked me. It was a question that lingered, even though the doctors had already removed it surgically.

It was all a mystery to me then, but now, with a deeper under-standing of cell regeneration and cellular memory, it makes perfect sense. Tracey wasn't just carrying the physical burden of a tumor; she was carrying the weight of life's many challenges. Raising a family of adopted children alongside her own, after believing she would never get pregnant, and managing the relentless crises that came with living in Africa—it all left its mark on her, physically and emotionally. In the final four weeks of the course, Tracey and I truly connected, spending time walking along the beach to and from our course location. We inspired one another to pursue our dreams with full force, each committed to improving the world. Tracey's vision blossomed into her healing non-surgical facility, an incred-ible achievement, especially as she balanced raising her family. Even when her husband was involved in a significant car accident, Tracey held onto her faith, believing in the greater good, and she turned her vision into reality. Tracey's healing non-surgical facility is a testament to her dedication, knowledge, and wisdom. Tracey is a remarkable practitioner with a vast heart and a true gift for healing.

47   UNKNOWN

The quiet storm

I had just opened my new clinic, a dream I'd nurtured for years. The place was buzzing with energy. I had three treatment rooms running, and the waiting list was growing by the day. Seeing so many people eager to change their lives on all levels was exhilarating—physically, emotionally, and spiritually. The clinic had become a healing sanctuary, and I thrived in the joy of helping others. One afternoon, a young couple booked a lymphatic drainage massage appointment.

They were quiet, almost reserved, as they entered the clinic. The woman had a hardened expression, a sourness that hung around her. She signed the intake form without a word, her face betraying a deep, simmering anger. I led her to one of the treatment rooms, trying to gauge her mood and the best approach to help her.

As we settled into the session, I gently broached the subject of breast cancer, a common topic for many of my clients. She revealed, almost offhandedly, that she'd had her left breast removed. Her youth struck me—she couldn't have been more than twenty-six. I began to share some insights, aiming to educate and empower her, but I didn't notice the warning signs that something was amiss. I was so focused on helping, on offering her knowledge and comfort, that I missed what she truly needed.

Fifteen minutes into the session, she suddenly bolted upright, her face contorted with rage. "Fuck this, fuck that!" she screamed, her voice filled with raw, unfiltered fury. "All I want is some peace, to stop the noise in my head!" Her words were like a storm breaking, and before I could respond, she was out the door, leaving behind a trail of anger and despair. She didn't pay, didn't say goodbye—just vanished as quickly as she had come.

I was left standing there, dumbfounded, with a heavy heart. I could not say or do anything to undo what had just happened. The clinic felt quieter than ever, and a lingering sadness replaced the energy that had once filled it.

I often wonder where she is now, whether she's found peace, love, or some semblance of happiness. Her pain was palpable, her anger a shield against a cruel world. I hope that wherever she is, she's found what she was searching for.

That day taught me a lesson I always carry with me: sometimes, the most potent healing comes not from words but from silence, from simply being present and offering a space where the storm can pass.

48   BITTER AND POOR ME

The lesson in miscommunication

It was a typical Monday evening when I revisited an encounter that would teach me a profound lesson about the power of words. I had seen this woman years before, and she had returned, booking an evening session after work. She struggled with weight, self-esteem, and the overwhelming demands of life. She came to me for a massage and guidance on a new path to better health.

As she lay on the table, enjoying the soothing strokes, we started a conversation about making positive changes. We discussed food intake, exercise, and the choices that led her to where she was. I intended to inspire and nudge her toward taking responsibility for her health. But then, in poor judgment, I said the wrong thing.

"It's all your fault," I said, referring to her struggles with diet and exercise. I meant to convey that our choices shape our health, but the words came out harsh and unfiltered. Once filled with a calming energy, the room exploded with anger. Her face flushed with emotion, and tears welled up in her eyes.

"I beg your pardon? How could you say that to me?" she demanded, trembling.

I immediately realized my mistake. "Oh, I didn't mean for it to come out that way," I stammered, trying to backtrack. But it was too late; the damage was done.

Her pain and frustration had been triggered, and she spiraled into a torrent of tears and self-pity. "It's not my fault," she cried, feeling unjustly blamed.

This moment was pivotal for me—a harsh reminder that words, even when well-intended, can wound deeply if not chosen carefully. I asked her if she wanted to end the session early, but she insisted on finishing the last fifteen minutes. We completed the session silently, and she left, her emotions still raw.

I thought the ordeal was over, but thirty minutes later, the phone rang. On the other end was her sister, her voice dripping with fury. She blasted me for my conduct, questioning my professionalism and accusing me of making her sister cry. She demanded a refund, refusing to hear my side of the story.

I took a deep breath, checking myself as I listened to her rage. "May I share my side of the story?" I asked, keeping my voice calm and collected, hoping to diffuse the situation. But my calmness only seemed to fuel her anger further.

"No, I don't want to hear your story!" she yelled. "All I want is my sister's money back."

And that was that. I refunded the money and never heard from either of them again.

This experience gave me a deep understanding of my responsibility in my work. It's not just about healing the body—it's about healing the spirit, too. Words are powerful, and in this case, they were my undoing. But every misstep is a lesson, and this one taught me to approach each client with even greater sensitivity and care.

49   JUSTINE

The healing path: Justine's journey to wellness

In early 2023, I received a call from Chris, my trusted hairdresser, while going about my usual day. He had a client in his salon, Justine, who had been captivated by the sign outside advertising "Lymphatic Drainage." Justine was in her mid-forties, vibrant but battling a persistent issue that had drained her both physically and emotionally—fluid retention. Once strong and agile, her legs had become swollen and tender, her ankles resembling overfilled balloons. The discomfort and distress were constant companions, and despite her youthful energy, she couldn't shake the fear that this condition might be permanent. Justine had recently embarked on a new journey with a multi-level marketing (MLM) business, fuelled by her passion for health and wellness. When Chris mentioned what I do, Justine's interest was piqued, sensing that perhaps this was the missing piece in her healing puzzle.

Justine and I began working together, and from the very first session, it was clear that her body was desperate for relief. Each touch and technique was met with a resounding response from her body as if it had been waiting for this moment to release years of accumulated tension and fluid. We explored not just the physical aspects of her condition but also the emotional and psychological burdens she carried. Justine, with her natural curiosity and drive, embraced the process wholeheartedly. She learned about the intricate workings of her lymphatic system and how it was linked to her overall health. We discussed her lifestyle, diet, and the importance of self-care, all of which played a role in her recovery.

As weeks turned into months, Justine's transformation was miraculous. The swelling in her legs began to subside, her ankles regained shape, and the tenderness faded. Justine was not just healing; she was thriving. She started sharing her journey with others, integrating her newfound knowledge into her MLM business and helping others understand the significance of lymphatic health. Her excitement was contagious, and soon, she was not just a client but a partner in spreading the message of holistic healing.

By the end of our time together, Justine had reclaimed her health and discovered a new purpose. Her experience with lymphatic drainage became a cornerstone of her business, inspiring countless others to seek natural and effective solutions for their health issues.

Justine's story is a testament to the body's ability to heal when given the right tools and support. She went from a woman burdened by physical discomfort and emotional distress to a beacon of hope for others facing similar challenges.

Justine's journey was not just about eliminating the fluid in her legs; it was about reclaiming her life, her confidence, and her belief in the possibility of complete wellness. Justine's transformation became a shining example in my practice, a story I would share with others who felt trapped by their health struggles. In the end, Justine did more than just rid herself of fluid retention—she opened the door to a new life filled with health, purpose, and the joy of helping others do the same. As for me, meeting Justine reinforced my belief in the incredible potential of the human body to heal and the importance of sharing that knowledge with the world.

50 CLAIRE

Claire's life had been marked by heartbreak and loss, culminating in a battle that would test the limits of her body and spirit. In 2023, Claire was in the intensive care unit, with doctors shaking their heads in defeat. They had run out of options; her condition was baffling. Claire was in excruciating pain—100 out of 10, as she described it. Each movement was agony, and her body seemed to be shutting down as if every system was failing all at once. Her daughter, Justine, was devastated, facing the unbearable prospect of losing her mother. Desperate for a miracle, Justine prayed fervently, asking God for a way to heal Claire.

Amid her despair, Justine received an unexpected phone call from a friend involved in a multi-level marketing (MLM) business. The friend insisted: "You must get your mum onto this stuff. It's a miracle in a golden bottle. It does not harm, and you have nothing to lose." With nothing left to try and every fiber of her being consumed by grief, Justine agreed. They had to do something— anything—to relieve Claire's suffering.

Claire took just two drops of the mysterious liquid in warm water. To their astonishment, her pain ceased almost immediately, if only for 20 seconds. Those 20 seconds were a revelation, a brief but powerful glimpse of hope that something more was possible.

But the story goes deeper. Claire's body was in turmoil, not just from physical illness but from an emotional wound that had never healed. Ten years earlier, she had lost her son, a tragedy that shattered her world. The grief she carried had become a cellular memory embedded deep within her body. This unresolved grief had weakened her immune system, making it impossible for her body to fight off infections and other health challenges. Her body was in complete meltdown, overwhelmed by the emotional and physical toll of her loss.

The "golden drops," as they would become known, worked miraculously. They didn't just address the physical symptoms; they calmed the storm of stress hormones that had been ravaging Claire's body. By reducing inflammation and allowing her body to relax, the drops gave her system the time it needed to repair and regenerate.

The courage to heal

When Justine reached out to me, her voice trembled with concern for her mother, Claire. She asked if lymphatic drainage could help, knowing that the golden drops had brought some relief, but Claire was still facing challenges. I assured her with confidence, "Yes, it will help." The golden drops had indeed made a difference, but Claire's tissues still clung to the deep-seated memories of her past, trapping waste that needed to be released. Lymphatic drainage was the only way to liberate her body from this burden.

As we began the treatment, I explained to Claire how increasing oxygen levels could awaken the body's innate intelligence, sparking the regeneration of her cells. It was as simple and profound as that. Reducing her pain could enhance her flexibility, dissolve her fear, and bolster her strength. The first time I saw Claire, I could see the struggle in her eyes. She could barely lay down, terrified that she wouldn't be able to breathe in that vulnerable position. I gently placed my hands on her, feeling the tension and fear that had gripped her for so long. "Your body knows how to heal," I whispered, "It's time to let go of the suffering and move forward."

With each session, Claire grew stronger. The physical relief was palpable, but something even more powerful was happening. She began to find the courage to forgive herself, to release the guilt that had weighed her down for so long. And in doing so, she rediscovered how to love—starting with herself. This is true healing: when the body and soul unite toward wholeness. Claire's transformation was a testament to the power of healing the physical body and the emotional and spiritual self. It reminded us that we create space for love, forgiveness, and life to flourish again when we release the past. Claire's story is a testament to the power of hope and the body's incredible capacity for healing, even in the face of overwhelming odds. It's a reminder that sometimes, the answers we seek come from the most unexpected places and that healing is not just about treating the body but also the deep emotional wounds we carry. This journey, beginning with a single drop of hope, would change Claire and Justine's lives forever.

51   SHIROMI

The mind–body miracle: Shiromi's journey to healing

Shiromi was a radiant woman with a smile that belied the pain she had carried for over a decade. For ten long years, she had endured severe neck pain and chronic headaches that robbed her of peace and joy. Like many others, she had seen countless specialists, undergone endless tests, and tried every treatment imaginable. But nothing seemed to work. Desperation led her to my clinic, a place she had heard about through a friend. I was her last hope. When Shiromi first stepped into my clinic, she bore the weight of far more than just her physical pain. An Indian woman deeply rooted in the belief that she must care for her family no matter the cost, she had endured years of silent suffering. A cancer diagnosis crippled her son-in-law, her husband was constantly traveling, and her relationship with her daughter was distant and strained. Despite the immense emotional burden, Shiromi insisted she was "healthy and happy." But the pain in her eyes told a different story: relentless sacrifice and quiet desperation.

As she recounted the countless visits to specialists and the futile treatments, I could see the weariness in her eyes. She had lost faith in the medical system, yet here she was, hoping against hope that I could offer her some relief.

As I began to massage Shiromi's head, I noticed something unusual—her skull felt misshapen, as though it had been molded by years of tension. This was more than just a physical anomaly; it was a sign of chronic stress. I explained to Shiromi that the shape of her skull reflected what was happening inside her body. The relentless stress she had been under had deprived her skull and the soft tissues surrounding her brain of vital oxygen. This had led to inflammation—a silent enemy wreaking havoc on her body for years.

Our sessions were non-surgical for the head, face, and jawline

In one session, Shiromi was free, and she couldn't believe it. Removing and slowly breaking the calcification released the inflammation and had immediate results, a truly remarkable therapy. Understanding the connection between inflammation and brain function was key to unlocking Shiromi's healing process. The brain, encased in the skull, is susceptible to environmental changes. When the body is under constant stress, it triggers an inflammatory response, which, in Shiromi's case, had settled between her skull and the soft tissues of her brain. This inflammation not only exacerbated her physical pain but also affected her cognitive functions, leading to memory issues, difficulty concentrating, and a general sense of mental fog.

I explained to Shiromi that her headaches and neck pain were not isolated issues—they were symptoms of a deeper problem. The chronic inflammation in her body was affecting her brain's ability to function optimally. This was why no number of painkillers or physical therapies had provided her with lasting relief. The real solution lay in addressing the root cause: the inflammation and stress that had occupied her body and mind. Through a combination of lymphatic drainage, non-surgical sessions, and stress management techniques, we reduced the inflammation in Shiromi's body. As the swelling subsided, her brain began receiving the needed oxygen. Slowly but surely, the pain in her neck and head began to ease. However, the healing process was not just physical; it was emotional and psychological as well. Shiromi learned to release the stress that had been suffocating her for years, and in doing so, she found herself again by breathing to relax. After many sessions, Shiromi's transformation was nothing short of miraculous. Her headaches and neck pain, once her constant companions, had all but disappeared. Her mind was more precise, her energy renewed, and her spirit lifted. Shiromi had not only healed physically but had also regained her sense of self-worth and confidence.

Shiromi's story is a testament to the incredible power of the mind-body connection. It shows us that true healing is not just about treating symptoms but understanding and addressing the underlying causes. Inflammation, stress, and the brain are intricately linked, and by recognizing this, we can unlock the body's natural ability to heal.

Shiromi walked out of my clinic a different woman—stronger, healthier, and more alive than she had been in years. Her journey reminded us that there is hope even in our darkest moments. When given the chance, the body and mind are resilient and capable of extraordinary healing.

This is the story of Shiromi, but it is also the story of countless others who have suffered in silence, unaware that their pain is more than physical. It is a story of hope, healing, and the incredible power of the human spirit.

52   TANYA

The healing journey: Tanya's triumph over alopecia

A struggle unseen

In the heart of Blackburn, 2019, Tanya walked into my clinic with a heavy heart and thinning hair. Diagnosed with alopecia, she faced the relentless challenge of female pattern hair loss (FPHL), a condition that strips women of their confidence and identity. Only in her mid-forties, Tanya felt the world's weight on her shoulders. The stress of a busy household, the pressures of a loving family, and the looming threat of Covid-19 all took their toll. She was booking an eight-week program at a hair loss clinic in South Yarra, desperate to slow down the inevitable.

Tanya's journey was more than just about hair loss; it was a battle against the internal and external stresses that had silently crept into her life. She wasn't just losing hair; she was losing herself. The hormonal changes, genetics, and underlying health conditions only added to her burden. But there was something in Tanya's eyes—a glimmer of hope, a belief that she could find a better way.

Tanya explored a different path by embracing the healing power of her own body instead of diving into the conventional treatments. She stepped into my clinic, not knowing what to expect but ready to embrace something new. She wasn't interested in massages, but the SOQI bed caught her attention. The warmth, the gentle rocking motion, the peace it brought her—it was as if she had found a sanctuary amid the chaos.

After just one session, Tanya felt something she hadn't felt in a long time: hope. The SOQI bed became her refuge, a place where she could escape the stresses of life and focus on healing. As the weeks passed, something remarkable began to happen. Her hair, which had been thinning for so long, started to grow back. The medications she had relied on were no longer necessary, and she felt an inner peace that she hadn't experienced in years.

But the most surprising change was yet to come. Tanya had a lump in her right breast, something her specialist had advised her to monitor. With the chaos of Covid-19 shutting everything down, Tanya had almost forgotten about it. As the world reached a standstill, she continued her sessions, feeling more energized and alive with each visit.

A transformation beyond expectation

Months later, as the world began to reopen, Tanya decided it was time to check on the lump in her breast. During one of her visits, she shared the news with me, her face alight with an energy I hadn't seen before. The scan revealed something astonishing—the lump was gone.

Tanya's transformation was nothing short of miraculous. She had lost 20 kg, her hair was fuller than ever, and the peace she had found within herself radiated outward. Tanya looked 20 years younger. Was it the lymphatic drainage, the weight loss, or the tranquility she had embraced? Perhaps all these combined worked in harmony to restore her body and spirit.

Tanya's journey didn't end there. She continues to visit me from time to time, seeking the regeneration she knows she can find. Her story is one of resilience, of choosing a less-traveled path and finding healing in the most unexpected places.

The power of belief

Tanya's story is about the power of belief—belief in oneself, the body's ability to heal, and the possibilities that lie beyond conventional wisdom. Her journey reminds us that sometimes, healing is not just about treating the symptoms but about finding peace within ourselves, letting go of the past, and embracing the future with hope. Tanya's triumph over alopecia is not just a story of physical recovery; it's a story of reclaiming life, one step at a time.

53 SUZIE

The healing spirit: a journey of devotion and transformation

Suzie's deep curiosity about the human spirit has always marked her life. Living in Melbourne, she had spent years searching for something that resonated with her soul. In July 2023, fate brought her to an event I organized for Darrell Wolfe. There, Suzie first heard about the incredible power of the human spirit and the healing abilities of the body's innate intelligence. Captivated, she felt an immediate connection to something greater than herself.

Her curiosity led her to book a stomach lift session, influenced by her best friend's glowing stories of its transformative effects. Suzie had no idea that this would be the beginning of a journey that would forever change her life.

From the moment Suzie experienced her first session, she was hooked. The experience ignited a fire within her—a desire to heal herself and learn how to heal others. Suzie immediately inquired about the courses I offered in lymphatic drainage and non-surgical healing.

With determination and passion, Suzie signed up for a course in Albury Wodonga, on the New South Wales/Victoria border, where I taught eight dedicated students, both men and women.

Suzie quickly stood out as a natural healer with hands that radiated unconditional love and care. Her thirst for knowledge was insatiable; she absorbed everything I taught with an inspiring and humbling intensity. Suzie's transformation from a curious seeker to a dedicated healer was miraculous. She spent hours practicing, learning, and perfecting the techniques, constantly pushing herself to understand and do more.

Her journey was not without challenges. Becoming a healer requires immense strength, courage, and an unyielding spirit. But Suzie was driven by something beyond herself—a calling to give back, pay it forward, and help others find the same healing she had discovered. Her devotion gave hope to her fellow students and everyone she touched.

Today, Suzie stands alongside me as a former student, fellow practitioner, and healer. Though she has not yet been trained as a non-surgical practitioner, it is only a matter of time before she achieves this goal. Her journey is far from over; it is just beginning.

Suzie's strength, courage, and unwavering determination have transformed her into a guiding light for others. She embodies the essence of what it means to be a healer—selfless, compassionate, and devoted to the well-being of others. Her story is one of transformation, of discovering one's true purpose, and of the incredible power of the human spirit.

The Healing Spirit is more than just a book—it is the power of devotion, the strength of the human spirit, and the transformative journey of one woman who found her calling and dedicated her life to healing others. Suzie's story will inspire millions, reminding us that we can transform our lives and those around us with courage, love, and determination.

54   DRUVIE

Druvie walked into my clinic with a serious back issue and a pain in the butt. He was a distinguished European gentleman, a corporate businessman in his late forties, who had dedicated his life to caring for his aging parents. They all lived together, and his commitment to his family and career left little room for a partner or a family of his own. The stress of balancing these responsibilities took a toll on his body—his back was seizing up, and his upper body was riddled with pain. Despite numerous scans and tests, the doctors couldn't pinpoint the source of his agony.

Eight weeks before a significant journey, Druvie came to me with a heavy heart. He was preparing to take his parents back to Europe for a wedding and a funeral. The irony felt like something out of a movie, but for Druvie, it was all too real. He was also anxious about leaving his two beloved German Shepherds behind and the toll this trip would take on his frail parents. It was a burden that weighed heavily on him.

When Druvie arrived at my clinic, he was desperate for relief—his last hope was to reduce or eliminate the pain that had plagued him for so long. After just one non-surgical session focused on his lower spine, he experienced immediate relief, something he hadn't felt in years. Over the next few weeks, Druvie continued with regular sessions, each one leaving him feeling more relaxed and at peace than he could ever remember. The transformation was profound. For the first time in years, Druvie felt truly at ease, and he began to understand that the key to his healing was the inner peace he was discovering.

This experience moved Druvie so much that he wanted his parents to feel the same gentle healing he had found. However, I never saw Druvie or his parents again after their European trip. People often don't come back in this line of work, and I might never see Druvie again. But maybe he no longer needs to see me—because he has finally found the peace that changes everything.

55 LUCY

The power within: transforming Lucy's life through oxygen

Lucy appeared to have a successful career, a beautiful home, a devoted husband, and a loving dog. Her life seemed picture-perfect, the envy of many. With her Italian sisters doting on her and a wardrobe full of designer clothes, Lucy embodied the image of a woman who had achieved everything. But beneath this polished exterior, Lucy was crumbling. She was a woman trapped in a relentless pursuit of perfection, burdened by the crushing weight of self-doubt and anxiety. Despite the outward success, Lucy felt she was never good enough.

Years of striving for an unattainable standard had severely affected Lucy. Her stress levels were off the charts, forcing her to rely on medication just to calm her frayed nerves. Her relationship with food became a battleground—oscillating between binge eating and starving herself, all in a futile attempt to gain control over her life. In reality, Lucy was spiraling into a state of chronic disease, her body and mind suffocating under the weight of her insecurities. The world saw her as a high-flying government official, managing immense wealth and power. But no-one knew the truth: Lucy was silently drowning in her fears, her breath shallow, her energy depleted.

When Lucy came to my clinic, she was exhausted, both physically and emotionally. She needed a way to escape the suffocating pressure of her life, to find a space where she could simply be herself. I knew that Lucy needed more than just relaxation; she required a profound transformation. The key lay in something as simple, yet as vital, as oxygen.

Oxygen is the life force that powers every cell in our body, fueling our vitality and clearing away the toxic waste accumulated from stress and poor health. Lucy's shallow breathing reflected her constrained life, which she barely survived. But by teaching her to breathe deeply and fully, we began to restore her oxygen levels, revitalizing her cells and reigniting her inner strength.

Her transformation was miraculous as she embraced the power of oxygen lymphatic drainage massage. The woman who once felt inadequate and defeated emerged as a powerhouse of confidence and vitality. Her stress levels dropped, her energy soared, and she started to see herself not as someone who had to be perfect, but as someone who was already enough. All it took was oxygen therapy and someone to hear her.

Lucy's journey demonstrates the incredible power of oxygen, not just as a physical necessity but as a source of profound healing and empowerment. By breathing deeply, Lucy reclaimed her life, transforming from a woman on the brink of collapse into a vibrant, powerful force of nature.

This is the story of how one woman's life was saved by the very thing that sustains us all: the power of oxygen.

56   LUCY

Breath of victory

Lucy's journey to true healing

Lucy was a fierce competitor—a young woman who thrived on the challenge of being the best. As a dedicated athlete and Year 12 student, she spent most of her teenage years in the gym, relentlessly pushing herself to excel in rowing and her studies. Yet, despite her impressive achievements, something was holding her back. Lucy struggled to breathe properly through her nose, a seemingly minor issue that would soon reveal itself as a significant obstacle to her success.

From the outside, Lucy appeared to be the epitome of strength and determination. She had a singular focus: to be number one in everything she did. Whether perfecting her rowing technique or hitting the books, Lucy was unstoppable. But beneath this exterior of invincibility, her body was fighting a silent battle. Lucy often found herself exhausted after intense training sessions, her muscles failing to recover. Nights were restless, filled with loud snoring, and a lack of energy marked her days. Despite numerous visits to specialists, no-one could pinpoint the problem. It wasn't until Lucy's mother voiced her concerns that a solution began to take shape.

Lucy's mother contacted me for advice after she worried about her daughter's constant fatigue and loud snoring. After learning more about Lucy's symptoms, I suggested a non-surgical approach targeting the root cause of her breathing issues. The plan was simple yet unconventional: open up Lucy's nasal passages and release the inflammation in her rib cage. This would allow oxygen to flow freely into her lungs, helping her body heal and recover as it should for a young woman in her prime.

At first, Lucy was skeptical. The idea of non-surgical treatment seemed far-fetched, especially when compared to the $6,000 surgery her parents had been considering. But with her mother's encouragement, Lucy decided to try it. The results were nothing short of miraculous. After just two sessions, Lucy experienced something she hadn't in years—a whole night of uninterrupted sleep. Her snoring ceased, and for the first time, she felt truly rested. The session was intense, with an hour of non-surgical work followed by another hour of rib cage release, but the payoff was worth every moment of discomfort.

Lucy's transformation was nothing short of remarkable. Not only could she breathe easily through her nose, but her energy levels soared, and her recovery times improved dramatically. She was back to dominating her rowing competitions, this time with the added strength of a body finally working at full capacity. The surgery that once seemed inevitable was now off the table, saving Lucy from unnecessary pain and future complications. Her parents were over-joyed, knowing they had made the right choice in avoiding a costly and invasive procedure.

Lucy's story demonstrates the power of listening to our bodies and seeking real healing solutions when traditional methods fail.

Lucy learned that true victory isn't just about being number one—it's about finding balance, health, and happiness. For Lucy, that victory began with something as simple as fresh air.

57   FRANCES

Unbreakable bonds: a journey of healing and resilience

The call for help

It was a quiet afternoon when my phone rang, the voice on the other end filled with desperation. Frances, a woman I'd never met, was pleading for help. She had suffered an extreme reaction to the Covid-19 vaccine, leaving her joints inflamed and her body wracked with pain. Her doctors were baffled, unable to offer more than temporary relief.

Frances had spent years as a caregiver for her husband, who had suffered a stroke in his early fifties. The stress of those years weighed heavily on her, a burden she had carried silently until her health began to unravel. Frances described how life had been good, how they had been happy. But beneath the surface, the stress of dealing with the pressures of everyday life had taken its toll, leading to his stroke and now her health crisis.

Frances had heard about my work with oxygen therapy and lymphatic drainage and how it had helped others recover from seemingly insurmountable health challenges. Desperate for relief, she booked an appointment for her husband first, jokingly calling him the "guinea pig." But as she spoke, it was clear that her situation was far from a laughing matter. Her husband arrived at my clinic first; his speech was slurred, his right arm barely moved, and his gait was unsteady. He had been under the supervision of a personal trainer, working out every other day, but his posture was off, and his lower back was stiff with calcification. His body needed more than just exercise; it required a comprehensive approach to healing. I started with a non-surgical lower back release to free up his pelvis, allowing him to walk straighter and more confidently. Over the following weeks, we strengthened his hamstrings, worked on his balance, and incorporated squats into his routine. Slowly but surely, his mobility improved, and his strength returned. The lymphatic drainage massage and SOQI bed sessions helped to relax his body, further aiding his recovery.

But as his progress continued, Frances's condition worsened. The pain in her joints was unbearable, and she struggled to keep working, the very reason Frances had taken the vaccine in the first place. The irony was not lost on her. Frances needed help, but the financial strain of medical bills and her inability to work left them with limited options. Despite this, I encouraged them to continue following my program at home, determined to see them through this challenging time.

Her husband's body grew stronger in a few short months, and his health improved significantly. Frances, despite her pain, found hope in his recovery. But her journey was far from over.

During one of our sessions, she mentioned her father, an older man who was facing health challenges. He walked into my clinic the following week, accompanied by his son-in-law. Frances's story was not just about her battle with pain; it was about the unbreakable family bonds, the resilience in the face of adversity, and the power of hope. Together, we embarked on a new chapter, extending the healing journey to another generation. Ultimately, it wasn't just about treating symptoms but about restoring lives, one step at a time. The experience with Frances and her family reinforced my belief in the body's incredible capacity to heal and the importance of a holistic approach to health. Their story is a testament to the power of perseverance, love, and the will to overcome even the most daunting challenges.

Epilogue: the legacy

Frances's journey, from the initial phone call to the recovery of her husband and father, became a cornerstone of my practice. It highlighted the need for a deeper understanding of health beyond what conventional medicine often offers. Their story inspired others, turning my work into a movement that emphasized the importance of addressing the root causes of illness, nurturing the body, and never giving up hope. Frances and her family became symbols of what is possible when we trust in the healing process, and their legacy continues to inspire countless others on their paths to wellness.

This book is dedicated to all who face seemingly insurmountable odds, but continue fighting for their health and loved ones, proving that the human spirit is unbreakable.

58   FRANCES AND JOHN

A heart's revival: the journey of Frances and John

John was a man of strength and resilience. Born in Europe, he arrived on foreign shores as a young boy, determined to carve out a life for himself. With hard work and dedication, he became a skilled concreter, laying down foundations not just for buildings, but for a future filled with promise. He married the love of his life, and together they raised two beautiful daughters. One of them was Frances, the light of his world.

For 60 years, John and his wife built a life of love, companionship, and unwavering support. They weathered storms together, constantly emerging stronger. But four months ago, John's world was shattered. His beloved wife succumbed to the adverse effects of the Covid-19 shot. The loss left John a broken man. The grief that engulfed him was palpable, and Frances could see her father slipping away, no longer the man he once was. John had begged his wife not to take the vaccine, but fear had driven her to make a choice that would tear their lives apart. Frances, too, was suffering. She had taken the vaccine because she needed to work, but the cost was severe. Her hands had become crippled, twisted into painful claws, and her body was ravaged with inflammation. Frances struggled to exist but had to be strong for her father and Adrian. The weight of her responsibilities was crushing, yet Frances knew she had to find a way to help her father heal.

John needed more than just physical care; he needed emotional healing, a release for the grief that was suffocating his heart. The non-surgical process required something even more delicate—mending a broken spirit. When I first met John, I was struck by the strength that still radiated from him, even in his pain. Frances's father was a gentleman, stoic on the outside, but inside, he cried out for relief. The day we began heart-release therapy was a turning point. As I worked to free the pain trapped in his body, the tears started to flow. John, a man of eighty years, apologized through his sobs as if ashamed of his vulnerability. But there was no shame in his feelings—only the raw, human need to heal. Session by session, we released the issues buried deep within his tissues, and slowly, John began to come back to life.

John's strength returned, not just physically, but emotionally. John started to see a future worth living, for his children and grandchildren. Frances watched in awe as her father, the man she feared she had lost forever, began to reemerge from the shadows of grief.

Twelve months later, John made a decision that filled Frances with a joy she hadn't felt in years. John had decided to return to his European hometown on a long-overdue holiday. It was a journey he had longed for, but had been too broken to consider until now. The decision was more than just a trip; it was a declaration of life, a choice to embrace the time John had left with renewed vigor.

As John prepared for his journey, Frances couldn't help but smile through her tears. Her father had chosen to live, to find joy again despite the immense loss he had suffered. And in his decision, she found hope for her own healing journey. John's story was not just one of recovery; it was the power of love, resilience, and the human spirit's ability to rise even from the deepest sorrows. Frances knew this was just the beginning of a new chapter for both of them. One filled with the promise of healing, hope, and the unbreakable family bond.

59 GAIL

The transformative power of lymphatics

Gail, a corporate businesswoman from Sydney, New South Wales, was always on the move, juggling high-stakes meetings and a demanding travel schedule. At 57, she was no stranger to the pressures of her career, and though she kept up appearances, the stress was beginning to take its toll. She had heard whispers about my "magic hands" and the healing power of lymphatic therapy from a colleague who had experienced a remarkable transformation after just a few sessions with me. Curious and skeptical, Gail looked me up during one of her business trips to Melbourne.

Gail wasted no time booking a 90-minute session, opting for the whole experience. "No point mucking around," she said with a determined smile as we prepared to begin. As the session unfolded, Gail was pleasantly surprised by the soothing, rhythmic flow of the lymphatic drainage massage. What she initially anticipated as just another wellness trend quickly became more profound.

By the end of the session, Gail was amazed at how calm and relaxed she felt, sensations that had become foreign in her high-pressure world. The therapy had not only eased her tension but also left her with an unexpected sense of lightness.

Intrigued by the immediate benefits, Gail decided to book a few more sessions over the next several days. With each session, she noticed subtle, yet powerful changes. The stress that had once knotted her shoulders began to melt away, and her skin, often dull from the wear and tear of her hectic lifestyle, started to regain its youthful smoothness. Most astonishingly, she noticed the bloating around her waist—a stubborn issue she had battled for years—was gradually disappearing.

As her energy levels surged, Gail felt a renewed vigor invaluable for her demanding career, especially the frequent flights that often left her drained. The transformation was undeniable, and it was clear that lymphatic therapy was more than just a temporary fix; it was a pathway to lasting health and cellular regeneration.

Whenever business brings her to Melbourne, Gail schedules a few sessions. These monthly treatments have become her secret weapon, helping her stay physically and mentally on top of her game. The once-skeptical corporate powerhouse is now a firm believer in lymphatic therapy, and she credits it with keeping her balanced, energized, and ready to face whatever challenges come her way.

60   LAUREN

Lauren's journey from pain to empowerment

Lauren was a dedicated professional working in the government sector, specifically in disabilities—a role that demanded both empathy and resilience. Her life was anything but typical. Diagnosed with multiple sclerosis (MS) in her early forties, Lauren had learned to cope with the chronic neurological disease that often left her feeling trapped within her own body. MS, the most common acquired neurological disease in young adults, had no cure and affected more women than men. Despite managing her symptoms, Lauren noticed a significant change when her stress levels spiked, making the disease more challenging to control. Her personal life added layers of complexity: she was caring for a foster child, dealing with a teenage daughter, and trying to support a partner battling alcoholism. Life was a constant storm, and the physical and emotional pain seemed to intensify with every passing day. Lauren's journey toward healing began when she decided to seek real medicine to manage her MS. She believed that the disease was more than just a physical ailment; it was deeply connected to the emotions she had buried over the years. The pain she felt in her shoulder and knees was a manifestation of these "issues in her tissues." Skeptical but desperate, Lauren started attending sessions designed to address both her physical and emotional pain. Each session was a revelation—she felt lighter, less burdened by the weight of her circumstances. The pain that once seemed unshakeable began to fade, replaced by a sense of calm and strength she hadn't felt in years. As Lauren's emotional state improved, so did her physical symptoms. The changes in her were so profound that they began to ripple through her family. Her partner, who had struggled with alcohol for years, started to show signs of transformation, becoming more present and supportive. Once distant and rebellious, her teenage daughter began reconnecting with her mother. Even the foster child in her care seemed to benefit from the newfound peace in their home. Lauren, who had once felt like a prisoner of her circumstances, was finally beginning to break free.

After a year of consistent sessions, Lauren's life had transformed in ways she never imagined possible. Her MS symptoms had significantly subsided, and the chronic pain that once dominated her life was now a distant memory. She no longer felt like a victim of her disease or her circumstances. Instead, Lauren felt empowered—more substantial and more in control than ever before. Lauren continued her sessions, now only once a month, to maintain her newfound sense of balance and well-being. Her story became a testament to the power of understanding the deep connection between the body and the emotions.

Lauren's journey proved that healing was possible, even for a condition as challenging as multiple sclerosis. The key was understanding why the body was flooded with inflammation and addressing the underlying emotional issues that fed the disease. Lauren's life had come full circle, from pain and despair to empowerment and hope. Her story inspired others facing similar battles, showing them that with the proper support and mindset, they, too, could break the chains of their illness and live a life of freedom and fulfillment.

61 TRACEY

Don't wait till you're diseased

The call came on a hectic afternoon, the kind where the weight of the world feels almost unbearable. It wasn't Tracey who reached out, but her partner, his voice trembling with worry. "Can you help us with Tracey's condition?" he asked, the desperation in his tone cutting through the silence. Tracey was suffering from an alarming amount of fluid around her waistline and chest, a sign that something was wrong. Alarm bells went off in my mind, and I could hear the fear behind his words.

When Tracey and her husband arrived, I saw the truth they had tried to conceal. Tracey was frail, her body ravaged by something far more sinister than they had let on. She was painfully thin, with fluid swelling beneath her skin. They had travelled an hour to reach us, likely hoping for a miracle. As I took one look at her, my heart sank. "Oh, my goodness," I whispered to myself. "This lady is not well."

After some coaxing, Tracey finally confessed. She had been battling breast cancer for four long years, the diagnosis coinciding with the onset of the Covid-19 pandemic. She had turned her back on conventional medicine, opting to forge her own path—a lonely road paved with pain and uncertainty. Her partner, a man worn down by grief, clung to her with all the love he had left, desperate to see her healed.

As Tracey spoke, I felt a deep sadness for the journey she had endured, filled with isolation and the firm belief that she could fight this battle on her terms. But that belief had come at a heavy cost. Her body was failing her, and the fluid that engulfed her was only a symptom of something far more insidious. Yet, amidst the sorrow, I knew all I could offer was hope and unconditional love.

I gathered my staff and decided that we would give Tracey a pampering day, a moment of respite from the relentless pain. Her partner, exhausted from years of care giving, needed this break just as much as she did. It was a small gesture filled with all the compassion we could muster. As I reached out to a colleague in town, I shared Tracey's story, knowing that her condition was beyond what I could handle alone. "She needs more help than I can give," I admitted, the weight of the situation pressing down on me.

The weekend with Lymphology Australia was a brief reprieve for Tracey. There was a glimmer of hope in her eyes, albeit faint. But the reality of her situation was impossible to ignore. The fluid in her body continued to accumulate, and it became clear that she would need it drained. As I watched her struggle, I couldn't help but wonder—why had Tracey waited so long to seek real medicine? Or perhaps, on some level, had she already made peace with the idea of passing on. The pain she carried was too deep, too all-consuming.

We never saw Tracey again after that weekend. Like so many others, her story became a haunting reminder of the fragility of life and the depths of human suffering. I often think about her, about the love her partner had for her, and the loneliness she must have felt as she faced her illness on her terms.

Ultimately, all we can do is offer what little we have—hope, love, and a belief that perhaps, in some small way, we made a difference. Tracey's journey may have ended in pain, but I hope that in those final moments, she found some measure of peace.

Her story stays with me, reminding me of the battles fought in silence and the resilience of the human spirit, even when all seems lost.

62   KAREN

The turning tide of menopause and chronic fatigue

At 57, Karen found herself navigating a challenging transition that left her feeling vulnerable. Her weight had spiraled out of control, a relentless force that seemed impossible to tame. Initially, Karen dismissed it as a typical symptom of menopause—a natural phase defined by the cessation of menstrual periods for twelve consecutive months, marking the end of her reproductive years.

Medically, menopause means the loss of ovarian follicles, the halt of follicular development and ovulation, and a significant drop in cyclical estrogen and progesterone production. These hormonal changes are well-documented, and Karen had expected to experience the common side effects: hot flushes, night sweats, and mood swings. Surprisingly, she had not endured the classic menopausal symptoms. Instead, her struggle was something more profound, more insidious.

Karen realized that her weight gain and other health issues were not merely the result of declining hormones but something more complex. She had been grappling with chronic inflammation within her immune system, a silent battle that left her feeling exhausted and unwell. It wasn't the usual menopausal turmoil; it was a condition that had been quietly undermining her health for years, and her issues in her tissues were the lack of love in her marriage and doing everything for her family, including working in the family business.

The real culprit was a chronic condition known as leaky gut. This medical term describes a compromised intestinal lining that allows toxins and undigested food particles to seep into the bloodstream. The resulting inflammation wreaked havoc on Karen's body, causing her to retain waste in her pelvic area. For years, she had lived with unexplained fatigue, persistent pain, and stubborn weight gain, unaware that leaky gut was the root cause.

Determined to reclaim her health, Karen embarked on a journey of discovery and healing. She delved into medical literature, consulted specialists, and connected with others who shared her struggles. Each piece of information she uncovered illuminated the intricate connections between gut health and overall well-being. She learned that maintaining a balanced diet, nurturing gut flora, and managing chronic inflammation were crucial steps toward recovery.

Karen's path was not easy. There were days of frustration and setbacks, moments when the weight of her condition seemed unbearable. But her resolve never wavered. She began to make changes—adopting a diet rich in anti-inflammatory foods, incorporating probiotics to restore her gut health, and practicing mindfulness to manage stress. Slowly but surely, she began to see improvements. The persistent pain lessened, her energy levels rose, and the unwanted weight started to diminish. Karen couldn't believe how lymphatic and non-surgical therapy could make such a difference so quickly.

As Karen progressed on her healing journey, she experienced a profound transformation. Her understanding of her body deepened, and she developed a newfound appreciation for its resilience. She realized that her condition was not a mere inconvenience, but a signal from her body urging her to make necessary changes and listen to its needs.

One evening, as the sun set and painted the sky with hues of orange and pink, Karen felt a sense of peace she hadn't known in years. She reflected on her journey—the challenges, the discoveries, and the small victories that had led her to this moment. Her transition was no longer a struggle but one of empowerment and renewal. Karen no longer saw herself as a label of chronic fatigue, but as a woman with issues she needed to resolve.

Karen knew that her story was far from unique. Many women faced similar battles, often dismissing their symptoms as inevitable parts of aging. By sharing her experience, she hoped to inspire others to look deeper, to seek answers beyond the surface, and to embrace the journey toward better health with courage and hope.

As the first chapter of her new life unfolded, Karen felt ready to face whatever lay ahead. She was no longer defined by her struggles but by her strength to overcome them. The turning tide had begun, and with it came the promise of a brighter, healthier future.

63 DONNA

The unexpected gift

When I met Donna, I felt a deep connection that would change our lives. It was the first lymphatic drainage course I'd ever run in the countryside of Victoria, Australia. Donna arrived three hours late, an older woman burdened with too much waste in her body and constant pain in her knees with fluid retention, which she thought was normal. Her energy was soft and calm, but there was something else—a quiet power that intrigued me.

As Donna settled into the course, listening intently to every word, I asked her why she was late. Her response was unlike anything I'd ever encountered, "I was scanning the frequency of the room and the people in it to see if there were any attachments hanging around," she said calmly. This admission caught me entirely off guard. Donna wasn't just an ordinary woman; she was a psychic medium, tuned into energies beyond our physical world.

That afternoon, after we'd finished the written work, I hesitated to work on Donna. Her pain and inflammation were palpable, but she also carried a heavy burden—one I couldn't quite define. Nevertheless, I began the session by focusing on her knees, reducing the inflammation, and then extending the healing to her entire body.

Donna had never worked with the lymphatic system before and had barely heard of it. But as we progressed through the course, something profound shifted within her. By the end of the three days, she had undergone a complete transformation—a 360 degree turn in her understanding of healing. She realized this was the key she had been missing in her journey to heal her body.

Donna's career had always been about helping others, connecting with the spirit world to offer guidance and solace. On the last day of the course, I asked her for a reading, hoping to connect with my triplet sister, Julie, who had passed away at 52. Donna agreed, and what followed was nothing short of extraordinary. "She has a lot to say to you, Michelle," Donna began, and for the next hour, we discussed Julie, my life ahead, and the path I was destined to walk. The experience awakened me and filled me with peace and purpose.

When Donna left that three-day event, she was a changed woman. Her knees were pain-free, and she was ready to continue her health journey with renewed vigor. But more than that, she had given me a gift—a connection to my sister that I had longed for, and a deeper understanding of the work I was meant to do in this world. This was the beginning of our journey together; one that would continue to unfold in ways neither of us could have imagined.

64   ANNA

Anna's awakening

Anna had always embraced her role as a healer. She was passionate about helping others on their journey to wellness. Her curiosity and dedication led her to constantly seek new and innovative ways to support the body's natural healing process. One day, while scrolling through social media, she discovered my course, and it immediately sparked her interest. It felt like destiny. Living in country Victoria, Anna didn't hesitate to book her spot and make the journey to Melbourne. She arrived with curiosity, eager to deepen her knowledge and understanding of the body.

From the moment we began, Anna was captivated. She was hungry for more and soaked up every piece of information. As part of the course, we delved into practical work, and during this hands-on experience, Anna confided in me about her lifelong struggle with her waistline—in her words, "the bane of her life."

A firm believer in the power of ice baths and spiritual practices rooted in nature, Anna knew this course was the perfect next step in her healing journey. She wanted to dive deeper and explore the body's capacity to regenerate and heal profoundly.

By the end of the second day, Anna's curiosity was piqued even further. She approached me and requested to experience a non-surgical treatment—specifically a stomach lift. As I worked on her middle organs and large intestine, there was an undeniable shift in energy. Anna felt something change, something she couldn't quite put into words. The scar tissue around her abdomen was released, and relief washed over her.

That night, Anna told me, she experienced something extraordinary. She visited the bathroom multiple times as if her body was purging itself of long-held toxins. More significantly, she had the best night's sleep she could remember. When she woke, her mind was sharp, clear, and focused in a way she hadn't experienced in years. It was as though a mental fog had lifted, and though she couldn't explain it, she knew something powerful had happened.

Throughout the weekend, Anna continued to receive sessions, each one deepening her understanding and love for the work. She embraced the teachings, applying them to herself and envisioning how she could help others.

Today, Anna is thriving. She has taken her newfound knowledge back to country Victoria, where she is fulfilling her passion as a lymphatic drainage massage practitioner. Her heart is whole, her purpose clear, and her love for healing has grown. The journey that began with curiosity has blossomed into a lifelong mission to bring wellness and transformation to those in need. And Anna, now more than ever, loves every moment of it.

65   LIZA

Liza was a beautiful soul, caught in a world she desperately wanted to control, yet was powerless against. Liza longed to transform her inner world, but in the process, she lost her grip on the outer one. Her first battle was with her eating and drinking habits—she was hooked on Diet Coke, a liquid acid that only served to deepen her pain. I understood her struggle; in my twenties, I was a binge drinker, too, trying to escape my inner turmoil. But while I could empathize with Liza's pain, I knew it wasn't hers to own. It was just a story, one we all have. But when that story lingers too long, it traps us in a grip that feels impossible to break. Liza's reality was tangled in a narrative that threatened to define her.

Liza had tried everything to lose the stubborn fat around her stomach, but nothing worked. Her joints ached constantly, and she felt trapped in a body that was betraying her. Desperate for a solution, she turned to a path she had never considered: lymphatic drainage and self-discovery.

The process was daunting, and the pain was real. The non-surgical stomach lift was particularly intense, sparking anger and frustration. Yet, Liza pushed through, trusting in the process. After just one session, the results were astonishing. The scar tissue in her lower abdomen, which had been holding her back for years, began to release.

Later, Liza reflected that the pain was worth it. Not only did she see her body transform, but she also felt a surge of new energy. Her sugar cravings vanished, and she embarked on a remarkable journey toward proper health and vitality. What began as a desperate attempt to lose weight became a life-changing experience, as Liza discovered a strength within herself that she never knew existed.

Liza's own words

I first met with Michelle in May 2023 at her Belgrave South clinic. I spent years suffering with a bloated stomach that looked like I was five months pregnant, and severe constipation. I had tried many home remedies, over-the-counter medicines, had CT scans, had colonic detox, once in Melbourne and once in Bali, and finally, a colonoscopy, which took me 12 months to get an appointment. Nothing came back from the colonoscopy apart from "you have a lazy bowel."

It was an ongoing battle that lasted for years; I felt helpless and depleted. I always felt flat and down, thinking I couldn't live with this forever, but I didn't know what to do. I didn't want to socialize as I always felt uncomfortable, and sometimes I would make up excuses not to go. I spoke to friends and family over the years, and they all had their remedies, concerns, and ideas, but unfortunately, no-one understood how I was feeling. It seriously can just take over your whole demeanor when you're feeling like crap all the time. I will admit my diet has been pretty bad all my life; I ate a lot of rubbish. Some days I could eat a whole block of chocolate. I drank v, diet Coke, lots and lots of coffee, smoked, ate junk food without even thinking about the effects this would have on my body and my health. I am not overweight, so I just ate whatever I wanted, including an earnest sugar desire. I am also on medication for depression, high blood pressure, and psoriasis. I have been on these medications for over 20 years, and I understand and appreciate this could have been contributing to how I was feeling; however, I wasn't going to stop my medications as I couldn't take any risks of spiraling further down the dark tunnel.

Last year, I started to think I had to do something myself. No doctor, medical advisor, or naturopath would do something to help me, and being a strong, determined 56-year-old woman, I thought it was up to me to find a solution.

I started researching on Google and found so much information on remedies, such as juice detoxing. You name it; I found it. I took a trip to Bali this year and found a fantastic masseuse. Gita asked me what I was here for, and I just blurted everything out, crying and telling her I just didn't know what to do. After my first session, she touched my soul and heart, and I could not believe she got it. We talked a lot about the lymphatic system. I had eight sessions with Gita during my holiday, and I will not say they were pleasant. It hurt like hell, I had bruises all over my body from the toxins and crap that were trying to get out of my body, and I cannot lie; I was starting to think I think I might have found something here.

Unfortunately, I still didn't go to the toilet regularly (maybe once a week or not), but I started feeling better when I was in Bali. I walked a lot, drank green juice, and ate Balinese jam. Once I returned home to Melbourne, I thought, "I don't care what this costs; I have to try and find a lymphatic specialist, as this had been the only thing that I felt in my heart could help me.

I started to research the effects of the lymphatic system, both negative and positive and slowly began to recognize that this could be the problem. Maybe my whole system was full of toxins and crap, and I had to somehow get it out without starving myself, detoxing, or just taking a tablet. One day, I searched for lymphatic treatment, and to my surprise, there was a clinic in Belgrave South. WTF? I immediately sent an email and explained my situation and what had been happening to my body. I received a reply within 5 minutes suggesting an appointment and offering a discount at a special price. I met with Michelle on that day, and Michelle explained what was happening to my body and the effects it was having.

Sometimes, I had no idea what she was talking about, but I just realized I did. We discussed diet, lifestyle, emotions, and attitude, and I thought, YES, she gets it... I believed in what Michelle was telling me, and I just had to believe in myself, my attitude and beliefs, and I had to commit myself. Luckily, I am strong-minded, and if I think in my head and heart, this will help; I am strong enough to commit.

Michelle went through the foods to cut out, introduced some lifestyle changes, and offered me treatment with the energy bed/ SOQI bed 3 times a week for 45 minutes. I am not going to say it was easy—no, it was not, but I had made a positive commitment to myself that if I didn't make these changes, I would either end up in the hospital again or live with this forever. Michelle, Judy and I worked together on this journey, and every time I walked out of the clinic, I just smiled and said, "thank god I met Michelle." I was starting to show vast signs of change. I was beginning to feel less bloated, more energetic, and less stiff, and sometimes I thought I had a skip in my step. Don't get me wrong, it's hard work; people are eating pizza in front of you, delicious cakes, roast potatoes, and my favorite, hot chips.

I still have a sweet tooth and probably always will, but I wouldn't eat a whole pack, or even a slice. During this treatment, I wouldn't say my constipation and impaction changed much. I was eating hemp seeds and chia seeds, and sometimes, I had to put a Movicol or two in my juices. This just seemed the only thing that would get me moving. I talked a lot about this with Michelle and every time I was having a treatment, she would kindly pop her head in and ask how my bowels are. You are doing so well, and you should be so proud she would say.

During one of our chats, Michelle suggested that she try non-surgical on my stomach, and I said yes, that would be fantastic. I went home and cried for her kindness and support. We started non-surgical; initially, it hurt, but it was certainly nothing to complain about. I could feel things moving, my tummy gurgling, and a slight popping feeling. WOW, this is amazing. I seriously could feel so much relief after only one session.

We continued with an energy bed and one non-surgical session weekly, and things started to move. I could feel Michelle's hands working the compaction around and breaking it up. I was so severely compacted that every time I went, I felt terrific, relieved, and so grateful to Michelle that she gave me 100% dedication and care; she had finally released all the crap that was being held in my body and not only was my stomach going down, I was using my bowels every day. I was happy to share my experiences and emotions with my family and friends.

In July 2024, I stopped my treatment as I went to Bali on holiday. I had massages with Gita again. It had been four years since my last visit. She asked me what I had been doing and was very surprised at how my whole body was accepting her treatment. I had no bruising or discomfort; overall, it didn't hurt.

I continue to empty my bowels every day, I have given up coffee (10 cups a day), and I continue to stay on track with my diet. I only eat gluten-free if I can, I juice every day, drink about 2 liters of water daily, and may have the odd hot chip or cake.

I will continue my treatment with Michelle once I have healed my broken knee and can drive. The treatment and support from Michelle has become part of my lifestyle, and I hope this story can help others as everything I have experienced and said is 100% from my heart and soul.

Thank you, Michelle and Judy xxx

66   TERESA

Teresa's triumph

In 2024, I met Teresa, a resilient cancer survivor who had undergone a double mastectomy, followed by breast implants. For years, she lived happily after her surgery, but then the dreaded news came—it was back. The cancer had returned. Teresa was determined to fight it again, and this meant enduring another round of aggressive drugs and treatments.

As time passed, Teresa noticed her right arm swelling, ballooning to an alarming size. The doctors had no clear answers and simply told her that it was part of the disease—a condition she would have to manage. But the swelling became more than an inconvenience; it was excruciatingly painful, rendering her arm stiff and immobile. Her specialist suggested she enroll in a clinical trial at Sydney University in New South Wales, Australia, which would cost her $10,000. Teresa was hesitant, unsure if the hefty price tag was worth it.

All Teresa wanted was for the swelling to subside and the pain to ease. I suggested she try just one session with me and see the results for herself. Skeptical but hopeful, she agreed. After that single session, her right arm felt noticeably softer, with a 90% improvement in movement and a significant reduction in pain. "Wow, wow, wow," Teresa exclaimed in disbelief.

Encouraged by the results, Teresa continued her weekly sessions with me. Before long, she could go on a much-needed holiday to Bali. She bought off-the-shoulder summer dresses for the first time in years—something she would never have dreamed of wearing. Her arm, once a constant reminder of her illness, was returning to normal.

Teresa canceled the expensive drug trial in Sydney. She realized that her path to healing didn't need to be filled with invasive treatments and unending costs. Instead, she chose to invest in her health in a way that allowed her to truly move forward, free from the burdens of her past.

67   SOPHIE

The breakthrough

Sophie had reached her breaking point when she called to make an appointment. "My legs are killing me," she said over the phone, "no matter what I do, I can't seem to strengthen my muscles. It's been years of this, and I can't take it anymore."

"Come in, and we'll figure it out," I replied, sensing the exhaustion in her voice. Sophie's frustration had built over time, but now the pain and swelling were unbearable. Years of searching for an answer had left her hopeless—until now.

When Sophie arrived, her legs were visibly swollen, and she moved with a stiffness that mirrored the tension in her voice. Sophie booked a series of non-surgical and lymphatic drainage massage sessions, and as we worked together, we uncovered layer after layer of underlying issues. It was clear that Sophie's condition wasn't just physical; her body had been holding onto something much more profound.

The root cause of her suffering came to light. Years earlier, Sophie had undergone full-leg laser resurfacing. What should have been a routine cosmetic procedure had turned into a nightmare. Her legs had developed extensive scar tissue, cutting off oxygen to the surface, and the accumulated scar tissue made her legs feel lumpy, painful, and perpetually sore. The scarring also affected her muscles, causing the constant weakness and pain she had been enduring for so long.

"Wow," Sophie gasped during one session. "I've been waiting for an answer for years. I had no idea it was all connected to the surgery."

But the physical aspect wasn't the only one we needed to address. Sophie's emotional state had taken a toll on her health. She felt disconnected from her work, lacked a sense of purpose, and felt like each day was an uphill battle. Her emotional blocks had compounded her physical issues. As a Lymphologist, I've seen this repeatedly—the hidden emotional self-talk, stress, and unresolved feelings that interfere with our cellular regeneration and healing.

Together, we embarked on a journey to heal Sophie's legs and free her from the emotional barriers keeping her from truly living. As the sessions continued, Sophie began to feel lighter—both in body and spirit.

This was more than just a treatment for her legs. It was a trans-formation, one that Sophie had been unknowingly waiting for. And it was only the beginning.

68 8-YEAR-OLD

The healing touch: a mother's desperate search for answers

I received a phone call one cold, dreary morning. The voice on the other end trembled with desperation. A mother, overwhelmed with fear and concern, reached out to me, her last hope. "Can you help my young daughter?" she pleaded. "The doctors have no idea what's causing her pain and discomfort."

Her daughter, once vibrant and full of life, was now reduced to a shadow of her former self, suffering from relentless stomach aches that had stumped medical professionals.

A friend had mentioned lymphatic drainage, a term unfamiliar to many but one that held the promise of relief. With hope in her voice, the mother asked if this mysterious therapy could be the answer. As she described her daughter's pain, my mind raced, searching for clues. I asked a simple question that led us to the root cause: "Is she having regular bowel movements?"

Her response, filled with uncertainty, made everything clear. The young girl, just eight years old, was not drinking enough water or consuming enough fiber—a common issue in today's fast-paced world where young people often neglect the basics of good health. This beautiful child, who should have been running, playing, and laughing, was consumed by stress. School, she said, was filled with bullies, adding an emotional burden that no child should carry.

I invited them to my clinic, where I spent 30 minutes performing a gentle lymphatic drainage massage around her waistline. The tension in her tiny body was palpable, but with each stroke, I could feel the knots of stress begin to unravel. She suddenly jumped off the table as I finished and rushed to the bathroom. Moments later, she emerged with a smile, her face beaming with relief—a significant bowel movement had brought her the comfort she had been longing for.

The transformation was immediate. The mother, overjoyed, watched as her daughter's pain vanished before her eyes. I took a moment to show her a few simple techniques she could use at home—golden rules that would ensure her daughter's continued well-being: more filtered water, more vegetables and fruit, and regular, gentle massages. With these tools in hand, the mother left confident and empowered.

I never saw the young girl again, but I didn't need to. The job was done. A life was changed, a child was healed, and a mother's heart was lightened. This story is not just about the power of lymphatic drainage; it's about the magic of listening to the body, trusting simple wisdom, and restoring health in the most natural ways.

69 JACK

A transformative encounter

The open day at my clinic was nothing short of magical. People traveled from far and wide, creating a vibrant atmosphere filled with curiosity and hope. It was a day of deep connections, where stories of struggle and healing intertwined. Among the visitors, one woman stood out—she approached me with a look of concern etched on her face, eager to talk about her 21-year-old son, Jack.

Jack had recently injured his elbow, and his pain was an excruciating 10 out of 10. A visit to the specialist, and an X-ray confirmed a minor hairline fracture, but the prognosis was disheartening. They told Jack they could do little except prescribe time off work—eight long weeks. As an apprentice, Jack found this news devastating. His daily routine came to a grinding halt; no gym, no work—just endless days of sitting around, feeling sorry for himself. Jack's mother, weary of her son's gloomy presence at home, wondered if there was anything I could do.

"Yes, of course," I replied confidently. "The great thing is, Jack is young, and his body can heal quickly with the right approach—lymphatic drainage massage and some non-surgical work. I believe one session will be enough for Jack to return to work pain-free."

Jack's mother was skeptical, but hopeful. "Really?" she asked, eyes wide with surprise.

"Absolutely," I assured her.

The following week, Jack came in for his appointment. I spent an hour working on his elbow and he spent thirty minutes in the energy SOQI bed. When the session was over, Jack left my clinic without any pain.

Curious, I asked Jack what his specialist had told him. "They said I'd probably need surgery down the line, and that medication was the only way to manage the pain. But honestly, the pain was more of a constant discomfort, a big pain in the butt more than anything else," he admitted with a grin.

To make matters worse, the doctors had sent a report to Jack's boss, mandating an eight-week break. Jack found the situation ridiculous but felt powerless to argue with his boss or the specialist.

As I watched Jack Walk out of my clinic, pain-free and full of renewed energy, I couldn't help but smile. Moments like these reinforced my belief in the body's ability to heal when given the right tools. And I knew, deep down, that this was just the beginning of many more transformative stories to come.

70   YOUNG GIRL

A new beginning at twenty-three

Imagine being twenty-three and having endured relentless pain every single month since you were twelve. What should have been the beginning of womanhood instead became a cycle of torment. Doctors labeled it endometriosis, fibroids, or pelvic inflammatory disease—clinical terms that did little to capture the reality of her suffering. This single mum had spent her entire young life battling this pain, determined not to continue down the same path. But where could she turn without relying on medication or facing invasive surgery?

Desperate for a solution, she turned to Google and stumbled upon my practice. The information resonated with her, and she felt a glimmer of hope—perhaps this was the answer this single mum had been seeking. We spoke over the phone, and I explained what was happening in her body. "It's inflammation," I told her, "flooding your pelvic area. When your period comes, the area becomes overloaded with waste. Your lymphatic system simply can't cope with it all, so some of it is left behind to fester, creating havoc in your bloodstream. This leads to a lack of oxygen and nutrients plus a build-up of scar tissue. Your body sends a pain signal, begging for relief, but conventional medicine doesn't know how to address it. It's no wonder you've been suffering." Her silent inflammation was because of the anguish over her parent's divorce and feels of guilt that it was her fault. The pain had become a cruel monthly ritual, a burden that would break even the most potent spirit. But there was another way. I introduced her to lymphatic drainage, a non-surgical approach that could offer her the relief she desperately needed.

In just one session, the pain she had endured for over a decade began to fade. It was nothing short of miraculous. Three sessions later, she was free. Free from the pain, the suffering, and the shadow that had loomed over her young life. At twenty-three, she had been given a new lease on life. How incredible is that?

71   LYDIA

Lydia's words

My journey to recovery

It is funny to revisit this story; it feels like it happened in another life, even to someone else, not just a year ago, to me. Things can change a lot in a year.

My sudden wake-up call

About a year ago, on one completely normal afternoon after work, I realized that my left leg was much more swollen than my right leg. I called a nurse and rushed to the emergency room. It was an enjoyable trip.

After a two-day hospital stay, they had no idea what was wrong with me. After that experience, I promised myself I would never walk into that hospital again.

A few days later, I saw my general physician, an old Serbian man who made me feel slightly better. Coming from my country, I knew he would be honest. I had so many blood tests and scans that, after 40 years of practicing medicine, he turned to me and said that, honestly, he didn't think he could help me.

There was even talk that I might have something in my brain, but with all scans and tests coming clean, all he could do was shake his head and wish me luck in finding out what was wrong.

Realizing I would not get anywhere with Western medicine, and with my discomfort and feeling my life span getting shorter, I started looking at more natural paths. One of them was acupuncture, which managed to help with the pain, but the swelling was still massively present. I had to quit work at this stage as I couldn't walk for extended periods. I was only 29 at the time; I thought my life, as I knew it with ease and without pain, was over.

Finding Michelle
While searching for other options, I asked many people if anyone had any suggestions. My friend suggested it could be something with the lymph node, so she told me to look online to see if I could find any lymphatic drainage clinics in Melbourne. After endless hours online with so many so-called experts and trials and errors, I finally saw Michelle, who was a Lymphologist doing lymphatic

drainage. Honestly, at that point, I didn't even know what that was or how that would change my life.

To this day, I am grateful for that random push to go exactly this way. I booked the appointment, and even after the first one, I knew I was on the right path and that Michelle was the person I was looking for. Just talking to her made me feel like I finally understood. It made me feel like she knew my challenges and how to help.

We did the first session, and she explained perfectly how my swelling started from all the stress during pregnancy, stressful jobs, and even childhood traumas that I kept running from and just trying to take care of everyone else. I was forced to take care of myself for the first time in forever and make myself a priority.

We went through each event and slowly discussed what happened. One thing I can tell you about Michelle is that you shouldn't come to see her if you are not ready for some harsh and blunt truths. More than once, she made me cry and accept that things happened that were not my responsibility and that I have other things to worry about now.

Some of the things that Michelle talked me through in our treatments were that we can't live in the past and that I need to put the past down and let it go so it doesn't keep catching up with me all the time and cause troubles in the form of mysterious disease and symptoms. Michelle taught me that I need to stop and be grateful for what I have today and appreciate how far I have come from a tiny village in Serbia to Melbourne, Australia.

I moved across the globe, alone, with only one suitcase and backpack, yet today, I have a family. I have a great husband, a *son, and another son on the way, as well as a great job that supports my choice to be a mother and a worker. One of the lessons I will always carry with me from Michelle is that I was, and am enough, exactly as I am.*

I don't need to be the best version of myself every day, I still matter. And as much as Michelle does physical work, her emotional work with me is much more critical.

Michelle saved my life.

Thanks to Michelle, my son today has a mother who is doing her best to break the cycles that have come before.

72　DANIELLA

The weight of pain and the quest for healing

Daniella's life was a testament to the unyielding grip of pain. In her late forties, her body was a battlefield—a relentless war waged by inflammation that ravaged her back, knees, shoulders, and neck. Each day was a struggle, each step a reminder of the agony that had become her constant companion. To make matters worse, the doctors had diagnosed her with depression, a label she had worn for twenty-five long years. The medications they prescribed offered little solace, dulling her emotions but never genuinely reaching the root of her suffering. Yet, Daniella continued to take them, trusting in the doctors' advice, even as quiet despair settled into her soul.

Her pain was not just physical—it was the echo of a childhood scarred by violence and rejection. Daniella's upbringing had been a nightmare. Family violence tore through her home like a storm, and her mother's cold indifference left deep wounds that never healed. She was a child, unwanted, a burden, and this pain followed her into adulthood like a shadow. When she became a mother herself, the cycle of torment threatened to repeat. Her heart ached for her son, but fear gnawed at her—fear that she would become the monster her parents had been.

Daniella made the agonizing decision to put her son up for adoption when he was just four years old. It was an act of love born from terror, a desperate attempt to protect him from the darkness that haunted her. She couldn't bear the thought of inflicting on him the pain she had endured. It was a decision that broke her heart but one she believed was necessary to save him.

Years later, Daniella's life was a testament to survival, but at a significant cost. The mind has a way of seizing control and reshaping reality, and in Daniella's case, it has built walls around her, imprisoning her in a world of fear and pain. The depression, the physical torment, the memories of a traumatic past—they all merged into a single force that ruled her existence.

But within her was a flicker of hope, a tiny, stubborn spark that refused to die. Daniella longed for something more—something beyond the pain and the pills. She wanted to heal, to break free from the chains that bound her, and to reclaim the life that had been stolen from her by circumstance and suffering.

I recount Daniella's remarkable journey of transformation, which healed her physical wounds and reshaped her entire life. I set Daniella on a 12-month intensive program, focused on weekly lymphatic drainage sessions designed to clear the deep-seated issues in her tissues, addressing both trauma and pain. Slowly but surely, Daniella began to transform.

When her mother passed away during this time, it marked a pivotal turning point—not a setback, but a powerful catalyst for change. In this moment of profound loss, Daniella put everything she had learned into practice, refusing to fall back into old patterns. Her determination to break free from her dependence on medication was unwavering. By the fourth month, Daniella had successfully weaned herself off all drugs, declaring she would never again rely on doctors.

This is the story of Daniella's journey. It led her to the brink of despair and back, challenging everything she believed about herself, pain, and the possibility of healing. It is a story of courage, resilience, and hope. Daniella's path was not easy, but it was hers, and in the end, it would take her to places she never dreamed possible.

73   CHRIS

Chris, a seasoned osteopath with decades of experience studying and treating the human skeleton, grappled with a mystery that his expertise couldn't unravel. At 56, his energy was waning, his get-up-and-go was gone, and his once-fit physique had given way to a hard, bloated waistline that refused to budge. Chris was at a loss despite his deep understanding of the human body.

His frustration led him to my doorstep after finding me on the internet. "Why am I struggling with my energy?" he asked, the concern evident in his voice. He was desperate to regain the vitality that had defined his younger years, but no amount of exercise or diet adjustments seemed to make a difference.

After listening to his concerns, I zeroed in on the root of the problem. "Chris," I began, "you need a non-surgical stomach lift to clear away the blockage of waste built up in your large intestines. This blockage is not only affecting your waistline but also causing you to wake up in the middle of the night to pee, interrupting your sleep and leaving you dehydrated."

His eyes widened in surprise. "How did you know that?" he asked, astonished by my insight.

"I just do," I replied with a knowing smile. Intrigued and hopeful, Chris booked in for three sessions of the non-surgical stomach lift. The transformation was nothing short of miraculous. After just one session, he returned the following week with a look of astonishment on his face. "I don't get up in the middle of the night anymore," he said, shaking his head in disbelief. "It's truly remarkable."

Chris's journey is the power of addressing the body's hidden blockages. His experience brought him back to life and reinforced that even the most knowledgeable professionals sometimes need a different perspective to solve their health mysteries. Through this transformative experience, Chris rediscovered the vitality he thought he had lost forever, and his story became another chapter in the incredible journey of healing that has touched so many lives.

74   MICHAEL

The day I met Michael

In early 2016, I met Michael, a man in his late forties whose life had been brought to a standstill by debilitating back pain. Michael had tried everything—physiotherapy, chiropractic treatments, and a host of other therapies—but nothing seemed to reach the root cause of his agony. His frustration was palpable, and I knew the solution would require more than physical adjustments. Michael's pain, like that of many others, wasn't just physical; it was deeply rooted in emotional turmoil that had been festering for years. In my experience, men often struggle the most with these issues. They're conditioned to ignore their feelings, to push through pain without addressing the underlying emotional blocks that exacerbate their physical symptoms. Michael was no different, but I saw a glimmer of hope in his eyes—a desire to change, to heal. I encouraged Michael to join my Pilates classes twice a week. I ran a thriving personal training business, teaching twelve weekly Pilates classes. Pilates is more than just a series of exercises; it's a powerful tool for strengthening the core and lower back, which, in turn, can alleviate a wide range of physical ailments. But I knew that for Michael, this was only the beginning.

In each session, we worked on building physical strength and the mental and emotional resilience he needed to confront the deeper issues. As we moved through the exercises, I could see the tension in his body slowly begin to release. It wasn't just his muscles loosening up—it was the emotional baggage he had been carrying for so long. At that point in my career, I hadn't yet delved into Lymphology, but my understanding of the body's emotional landscape was already deeply ingrained in everything I did. I knew that true healing required addressing the whole person—mind, body, and spirit. For Michael, this holistic approach was a revelation. As he strengthened his body, he also began to improve his mind, gradually chipping away at the emotional blocks that had kept him in pain for so long. By the time we finished our work together, Michael wasn't just free from pain—he was different. His journey was a powerful testament to the idea that healing is possible when we address the root causes of our suffering, not just the symptoms. And for me, it was another reminder of the transformative power of my work. This was just one of the 100 case studies that would shape the foundation of my future work in Lymphology. Like so many others, Michael's story reaffirmed my belief that the key to healing lies in understanding the complex interplay between our physical bodies and emotional well-being.

75   JO'S DAUGHTER

After her session, Jo was overwhelmed with joy. With a bright smile, she turned to me and asked, "Will this help my daughter's nose?"

"Okay, Jo, what's been going on with your daughter?" I replied.

Jo took a deep breath and shared her story. When her daughter was a teenager, she was struck in the nose by a basketball, leaving her struggling to breathe ever since. Now, at 24 years old, her daughter still faced the aftermath of that accident. Specialists had suggested surgery, but Jo was hesitant. The path to surgery was uncertain—there was no guarantee it would make a difference, and being a cosmetic procedure, it was also costly.

I met Jo's daughter the following week and conducted non-surgical sessions on her nose and face. The treatment cleared her sinuses and unblocked her nasal passages, allowing more oxygen to flow and promoting healing. Remarkably, her nose appeared straighter after just one session. Jo and her daughter watched in awe, unable to believe the transformation. Now Jo's daughter was breathing better.

"I can't believe it worked so quickly," Jo exclaimed. "One session, and you're breathing better and looking straighter. It's amazing!"

Jo's gratitude was palpable. The non-surgical approach improved her daughter's breathing and restored her confidence. We celebrated this unexpected breakthrough together, hopeful for the future and possibilities ahead.

76   MARK

A shared passion: how the course run by Michelle brought us closer together

I was initially drawn to the lymphatic drainage massage course because of my wife's interest, but I quickly discovered my passion. The three-day course was thoroughly enjoyable and eye-opening. Not only did I gain valuable skills, but I also found myself eager to support my wife in setting up her business. The course Michelle Richardson ran exceeded my expectations, and I'm grateful for the knowledge and experience I gained. I highly recommend it to anyone interested in lymphatic drainage massage.

Mark Quirk
Thurgoona, NSW

77   SHARON

In the early days of my lymphology work, I was invited to give a talk in Albury, Australia. As I stood before the audience, one person stood out—Sharon. Sharon had been a dedicated schoolteacher for most of her life and had always cared deeply for others. Still, the challenges of the Covid-19 pandemic had ignited a desire within her to make an even more significant impact. She was searching for a new direction, a way to transform lives.

After the talk, Sharon approached me with an idea. She proposed hosting a weekend workshop in Albury, eager to learn more about lymphatics and explore how it could change the course of her life and the lives of others. This marked the beginning of Sharon's remarkable learning, growth, and profound transformation journey.

Sharon's journey—a life of purpose: my journey to becoming a lymphatic drainage Therapist

Discovering the power of lymphatic drainage massage

Curiosity has always been a driving force in my life, and one day, I found myself fascinated by the intricacies of the human body's lymphatic system. How does it work? What role does it play in maintaining optimal health? My quest for knowledge led me to a life-changing opportunity: a lymphatic drainage massage course taught by the renowned Michelle Richardson.

As I enrolled in the course, my excitement grew. I was eager to delve into lymphatic health and understand its significance. Michelle's expertise and passion were palpable from the start, and I was impressed by the depth of knowledge she shared with us. The hands-on experience was invaluable, allowing me to grasp, and confidently apply the techniques.

The course was a revelation. I learned how the lymphatic system, often overlooked, plays a vital role in our body's defense and detoxification processes. By stimulating lymphatic drainage,

I could help individuals boost their immune function, alleviate chronic pain and inflammation, and even support cancer recovery. The potential to empower people to take control of their health was exhilarating.

Michelle's dedication and passion were contagious. Her teaching style was engaging, informative, and inspiring, making complex concepts accessible to all. Her expertise and experience shone through in every aspect of the course, from the comprehensive manuals to the guided practice sessions.

As I completed the course, I knew I had to share this knowledge with others. I invested in the necessary equipment and transformed a space in my home into a serene and welcoming environment for clients. With Michelle's guidance and encouragement, I began building my business, eager to spread the benefits of lymphatic drainage massage.

The response has been remarkable. Clients from diverse backgrounds and age groups have sought my services, seeking relief from various health concerns. Witnessing the positive impact on their well-being has been incredibly rewarding. I have seen individuals regain energy, experience reduced swelling and pain, and even report improved mental clarity.

Michelle's course has been a catalyst for my journey. Her tireless efforts to educate and inspire have created a ripple effect that extends far beyond the classroom. I'm grateful for her mentorship and the opportunity to make a meaningful difference in people's lives.

As I continue to grow my business and share the benefits of lymphatic drainage massage, I remain committed to Michelle's high standards of excellence. Her legacy lives on through the countless lives touched by her teaching, including mine.

Sharon Quirk
Thurgoona NSW

78   SANDRA

My healing journey started around May 2023, when I was feeling overwhelmed, fat, frumpy and generally out of sorts. Not the 'normal me.' Physically, I felt like I was a lot older than I was. I was so down and depressed that when people spoke to me, I would cry (at the drop of a hat)—for no reason and with no control whatsoever. This wasn't me—I'm usually upbeat, happy, healthy and sociable! I'm no spring chicken, but I do pride myself on exercising regularly, keeping healthy and busy. The way I was feeling was not usual, and I didn't like it. I didn't want to continue feeling horrible, but I also didn't know what to do. I thought I would be stuck with this feeling for the rest of my life—that this is what it will always be.

From the beginning, Michelle shared with me and asked me to say the following to myself anytime I was feeling low: 'I am healed! I am loved! I am a brave heart. From the moment I open my eyes to the minute I close my eyes each day I WILL honor, love, and respect myself and others!" WOW!! What a powerful phrase to confirm with yourself and remind ourselves of who we are and that we are essential in this world!

Before, feeling inadequate and out of sorts, I walked daily (at least 8–10 km) and generally felt well for my age. I currently hold down jobs, and understandably, I often get tired for that very reason, but, for my age, people are astonished that I do what I do. As an Executive Assistant, I work in an office at a desk, but I also do shift work on my feet for hours in hospitality, customer service, and retail.

My introduction to lymphatic drainage/massage started one day in late April/early May last year, when I was working in my office in the Melbourne CBD. I caught up with a fellow worker who I hadn't seen for a while for a coffee. She instantly knew I wasn't my usual optimistic self—something was wrong. My demeanor was very low; I was sad, and she was worried about me and didn't like what she saw.

On explaining to her how I was feeling (and breaking down crying), she took my hand and shared with me her experiences with lymphatic drainage/massage and the positive healing results she had experienced from her treatments. This lady has been through a lot of medical challenges over the years—including difficulty walking. Still, she has found so much positivity and relief in her condition by having lymphatic sessions. She suggested I go back to my desk and Google my nearest lymphatic drainage person, make an appointment, and give it a go. I had nothing to lose and lots to gain!

I wasn't prepared to continue feeling like this (it was horrible, and I didn't like it), so I looked up Michelle Richardson's Energy Wellness lymphatic drainage massage and SOQI bed in Belgrave South (close to home) and made an appointment. I was unsure what was in store, but I was willing to take the chance!

At my first appointment, Michelle assured me that she could help. She put my mind at ease and gave me hope but emphasized that it would not happen overnight!

We must remember that one consultation will not fix everything and that the session needs to be combined with helping ourselves repair our bodies. The process allows us to self-heal ourselves through attitude change and understanding how we approach our ailments.

Michelle told me about the four laws of health:

1. Breathing.

2. 'Plant-based' food (no processed , i.e. dairy).

3. Be aware of mental & emotional stress;

4. Belief system

'Controlled' Breathing—Wow! It's something I've thought about for years—how it can calm you, help you through pain, anxiety, etc., but I never followed through with it. When I feel something building that could cause me stress, I go through my deep breathing routine—things look so much calmer, clearer and more logical on the other side. Breathing is an integral part of helping heal ourselves—it works wonders, and we do it every day—breathe!!

As I had further consultations with Michelle, I felt much better, and my mindset changed in many ways. With my positive attitude and a new way of thinking, I welcomed back the real 'me'! Concentrating and being aware of our mental and emotional stress is another way to self-heal ourselves. We all know how stress can impact our health—both mental and physical, churning us inside and out, headaches, anxiety, etc. Concentrating once again on 'breathing' through the situations truly helps—but no-one can do this but us; we need to help ourselves.

At my many sessions with Michelle, there were often challenges along the way. Michelle would share her wealth of information on 'how the body works,' what triggers this, and what aggravates that! Michelle would also explain how the lymphatic system works, why and how things happen, and what happens if you do something or if you don't do something—all things that I needed to take on board to assist me in healing my own body. This valuable information helped me on my road to recovery and getting back to normal.

After 3–4 sessions, I was beginning to feel my old self again—energy levels were back, bloating, sluggishness and overall 'low' feelings were gone and life was looking much better! As each treatment came along, I felt better—I had changed my mindset and begun exercising again, eating correctly, and drinking the necessary water to help the body function properly. I was returning to my old 'positive' self; that horrible initial feeling of being unwell was gone. My mental attitude had changed in what I thought and did; with this mindset, my general well-being returned.

Certain areas of my body needed more work, and often, working and concentrating on these areas in the session caused pain. However, the discomfort was necessary to release/move or break up the blockage or scar tissue causing the problem. The pain was for a good reason, and my controlled breathing got me through it.

Currently, I have fortnightly consultations with Michelle, and whilst there are weeks when I just need a general well-being massage, there are still other weeks when I may have a minor niggle or a particular area that needs working on. Sometimes, it could just be a sore neck from sleeping wrong or a slightly sore back from sitting at my desk too long. Either way, I leave my treatment feeling relief, so much more comfortable and floating on air!

The medical system in the 21st century (through drugs and often surgery) is not always the answer. We need to open our minds and look at other non-surgical treatments and options out there that can provide similar, if not better results without the costly use of 'cover-up' drugs. Changing our attitude and understanding that we can heal ourselves opens up many new options to improve our health 'naturally'!

Initially, on a couple of occasions, I would mention to Michelle I was thinking of going to the doctor—but she has always reassured me that, with positive thinking and taking on the 'healing ourselves' attitude, we don't need 21st-century drugs or medication. Deep, controlled breathing through pain and stress has worked wonders for me. I've even been able to go off my blood pressure tablets through my controlled breathing process, and my doctor is astounded. Breathing relieves my stress and anxiety.

The great feeling I get from having a lymphatic drainage massage (and Michelle's words of wisdom and healing hands) is just wonderful. I can't thank my fellow worker enough for recommending this treatment. Of course, I can't thank Michelle enough—she has an immense wealth of knowledge on the lymphatic system (which she shares with me). She is willing to listen and encourages me to continue healing on this positive journey.

I could go on for a lot longer, telling you about the positivity I feel after consultation with Michelle; however, in the interest of allowing others time and space to tell 'their' story, I'm happy to sum up my experience as follows:

People I interact with regularly have noticed a change in me and reached out to find out what I've done. Whenever I get the opportunity (and often make it happen anyway), I praise Michelle's lymphatic treatments and recommend her to as many people as possible.

I'm living proof of how these treatments can change your life, and I want to share it with others who may be going through the same feelings and health issues that I initially experienced.

IT WORKS! Michelle is 'great' at what she does, and I'm so glad I found her to help me!

79   AMAZING WOMAN

The awakening of an amazing woman

A woman of profound grace and quiet strength, was not just any beauty therapist. Trained in the delicate art of natural healing, she had mastered various therapeutic modalities, blending ancient wisdom with modern techniques. Her career was a tapestry of rich experiences. Yet, despite these varied pursuits, this amazing lady felt an unshakable yearning—a desire to deepen her understanding of the human body and its incredible capacity for healing.

This quest for knowledge led her to my sessions, where this amazing lady sought to learn the transformative power of lymphatic drainage. We had an unspoken connection that transcended the ordinary from our first meeting. Perhaps her middle name, Julie, resonated deeply within me, or maybe it was her unwavering belief in the body's ability to heal itself. Whatever the reason, our bond felt pre-destined, as if our paths were meant to cross in this life.

But beneath her poised exterior lay a heart heavy with sorrow. The world had changed in ways she could scarcely comprehend, and the Covid-19 mandates had left her reeling. She was bitter, lost, and grappling with an overwhelming sense of betrayal. Friends she once held dear had drifted away, consumed by a world that seemed to have fallen under the spell of greed and destruction. The pain of losing her daughter, coupled with the erosion of once-cherished relationships, left Catherine in a state of despair, her spirit wounded and her trust shattered.

This amazing lady's body, too, bore the weight of her emotional turmoil. Anger and heartache had taken their toll, allowing toxins to fester within her, poisoning her from the inside out. It was clear that she needed more than just physical healing; she required a deep cleansing of her mind, body, and soul. Many people fail to realize the insidious nature of such internal waste—how it quietly erodes health, saps vitality, and destroys lives from within. As we began her treatment, I could see the layers of pain and bitterness start to peel away. This amazing journey toward healing was not just about removing the physical toxins; it was about reclaiming her sense of self and rediscovering the joy and peace buried beneath years of hurt. She was determined to break free from the chains of anger and despair, to purge the darkness that had taken root within her, and to emerge stronger, more resilient, and more at peace with the world around her.

This was just the beginning of her journey of transformation, healing, and, ultimately, redemption. Little did she know that her story would inspire countless others and be a beacon of hope in a world that desperately needed it.

80   SAMANTHA

In a heartwarming turn of events, one of my clients shared the story of her dear friend, Sam, who had been suffering from excruciating pain in her elbows. Sam was on the brink of turning 60 and had begun visiting numerous specialists who all diagnosed her with arthritis and tennis elbow, insisting that she would need to manage the pain with drugs for the rest of her life. But Sam, full of life and spirit, refused to accept this fate. "I'm too young to be crippled by this," she told me. "I've heard you work miracles."

I smiled, knowing that the true miracle lies within each person. Something extraordinary happened in just one lymphatic drainage massage session: the pain that had haunted Sam for so long vanished. Even I was taken aback by the rapid transformation. Sam was overjoyed and beyond grateful that her friend had led her to me when she felt lost and desperate.

Sam visits monthly for maintenance and a friendly chat to ensure her body stays balanced. She still finds it hard to believe that her pain is gone, but the relief she feels is undeniable. This journey with Sam is a testament to the power of the body's ability to heal when given the proper support, and it's stories like hers that inspire me to continue this incredible work.

81   JOUMANA

The journey of healing

Joumana, a vibrant woman from Sydney, New South Wales, discovered my work through social media. She was captivated by the stories of recovery and the non-surgical methods I employed. Joumana saw an opportunity as a mother to a daughter deeply entrenched in beauty therapy. She believed that adding lymphatic drainage to her daughter's skillset could enhance her practice and provide a profound way to heal emotional and physical pain. Driven by curiosity and a desire to empower her daughter, Joumana reached out to me. Together, they enrolled in my three-day workshop, a decision that would transform their lives. Neither of them had any prior experience with lymphatic drainage, but they were eager to learn. The workshop was structured to include practical sessions each afternoon, where participants could practice with one another.

During these sessions, something remarkable happened. Joumana's daughter, who believed she was in perfect health, began to experience profound shifts. She was stunned by the revelations that surfaced; issues she had never been aware of yet, they had been festering beneath the surface for years. It was a powerful reminder that our physical ailments often have deep-rooted emotional origins, lying dormant until the right moment reveals them.

As the workshop progressed, it became clear that this was not just a new skill for Joumana's daughter, but a journey of self-discovery and healing. Realizing that her inner world had impacted her physical health was eye-opening. By the end of the three days, she was equipped with a new therapeutic tool and a deeper understanding of her body and mind.

Since then, Joumana's daughter has integrated lymphatic drainage into her beauty practice in Sydney, and the results have been extraordinary. Clients are looking better and feeling better as they release long-held emotional pain. Joumana is immensely grateful that her daughter chose to embark on this journey, recognizing that this newfound knowledge likely prevented more serious health issues.

This chapter of their lives is a testament to the power of awareness and proactive healing. What began as a simple interest in a new skill became a profound journey of transformation, impacting not just their lives, but the lives of everyone they touch through their work.

82   BELINDA

Belinda's transformation

Belinda had been suffering for years with pain that seemed to have settled in every corner of her body. It was the kind of relentless discomfort that she had resigned herself to live with, thinking it was just something she had to endure for the rest of her life. Like so many others, Belinda believed that her pain was an inevitable part of aging, something that could only be managed, but never truly healed.

Then, one day, while chatting with a close friend, the topic of lymphatic drainage came up. Her friend had recently seen me for treatment and couldn't stop raving about the results. Belinda had heard whispers about this therapy before but had never given it much thought. The idea seemed too simple, too good to be true. After all, if it worked, why didn't everyone know about it? But her friend was persistent. "What do you have to lose?" she said. "It's just a small investment in your health, and who knows, you might find yourself living pain free."

Intrigued but still a bit skeptical, Belinda decided to give it a try. She booked an appointment, unsure of what to expect but hopeful that this could be the answer she had been looking for.

When she stepped into the clinic, Belinda felt a sense of calm and care that she hadn't experienced in any other medical setting. I educated her on how the lymphatic system works and its impact on the body, opening her eyes to a new understanding of health. She realized that her body wasn't just breaking down; it was calling out for help.

During the session, we worked together to gently heal her body, addressing the root causes of her pain. The experience was nothing short of transformative for Belinda. She left the clinic feeling lighter, both physically and emotionally. When Belinda returned the following week, she could hardly believe the change. Her body was 95% pain-free. She had achieved this without the need for drugs, without invasive surgery, and with a newfound knowledge of how to take care of herself. Her joy was palpable.

As part of her healing journey, we focused on small but impactful changes—drinking more water, reducing sugar intake, and maintaining a positive mindset. Belinda embraced these adjustments enthusiastically, feeling empowered by the understanding that she could influence her health.

Today, Belinda is a different person. The pain that once defined her life is now a distant memory, replaced by a sense of well-being and happiness that she never thought possible. It all started with a simple decision to invest in herself, to believe that healing was possible, and to take that first step towards a pain-free life.

83   LORETTA

Loretta's journey—the hidden cost of perfection

Loretta was a stunning young woman who dreamed of achieving the perfect body. Her vision led her overseas for a procedure she believed would quickly fix her insecurities. Like many young women, she was lured by the promise of beauty, convinced that a slim figure would bring her happiness and self-worth. But what she didn't anticipate was the price she would pay—one far greater than the thousands she spent on surgery.

The physical pain was intense, but it was the emotional turmoil that trapped Loretta in a cycle of self-loathing. Surgeons often fail to explain the full scope of the recovery process—the agonizing pain, the potential for lifelong complications, and the deep scars left not just on the body but on the soul. They focus on the external transformation, neglecting the internal wounds that can linger long after the incisions have healed.

For Loretta, the journey to what she thought would be her dream body turned into a nightmare. The mirror still reflected her beauty, but in her mind, the image was distorted by the trauma of her experience. Hours of lymphatic drainage massage became her solace, slowly releasing the physical pain and the emotional burden she had carried since the surgery.

In time, Loretta found comfort again. But the lesson she learned was profound. She confided in me, sharing that if she had known the extent of the pain and the long, grueling recovery, she would never have undergone the procedure.

Many overlook Loretta's discovery: if you cannot see the beauty within, no amount of work on the outside will ever change the way you see yourself. The fundamental transformation begins with self-acceptance, not with a surgeon's knife.

84   SIMONE'S PARTNER

The healer within

Simone had always been a vibrant, energetic woman, but over the years, she had battled a stubborn waistline that refused to budge. She had tried everything, from strict diets to grueling workout regimens, yet nothing seemed to work. Frustrated and desperate for a solution, Simone journeyed from Sydney to Melbourne to see me, intrigued by the energy bed I had been showcasing on social media. She hoped that this unconventional method would finally be the answer to her prayers.

When Simone arrived at my clinic, she was both hopeful and skeptical. As she lay on the energy bed, I could see the tension in her body, the years of frustration etched into her face. But as the session progressed, something remarkable began to happen. Simone's body started to relax, and she could feel the gentle, healing energy working through her. By the end of the session, she was amazed at the difference she felt—not just in her waistline but in her overall sense of well-being.

Simone was so impressed with the results that she couldn't wait to share her experience with her partner. He had been suffering from excruciating knee pain for over 20 years, a consequence of his days as a professional soccer player. Despite seeing some of the top chiropractors and specialists in the world, his pain persisted, and it was taking a toll on his quality of life. Encouraged by Simone's enthusiasm, he visited me to see if I could help where others had failed.

When he arrived, I could see the weariness in his eyes, the burden of years of pain and disappointment. As we talked, I shared with him my belief that the root cause of his inflammation and knee pain wasn't just physical—it was deeply connected to the immense stress he was under in his high-pressure career. The demands of his job had been relentless, and his body was crying out for relief. I warned him that if he didn't slow down and address the stress in his life, the consequences could be far worse than just painful knees.

As the session began, I focused on helping him release the tension and stress that had built up over many years. By the end of the session, he stood up, and a look of astonishment crossed his face. The pain that had plagued him for two decades had suddenly vanished. "Wow," he exclaimed, "I've seen some of the top specialists in the world, and none of them could do this. The pain is gone."

He paused as if processing the significance of what had just happened. Then he looked at me with a newfound understanding and said, "The healer is within."

In that moment, he realized what I had known all along—that true healing comes from within and that the body can heal itself when given the proper support and care. This revelation was just the beginning of his journey to a healthier, pain-free life, and it marked the start of a profound transformation that would change his life forever.

85   ELLEN

Ellen's race to renewal

Ellen was the embodiment of vitality. A fit and active professional who firmly believed in the power of self-care and the importance of nurturing a healthy relationship with oneself. As a single mother of two young children, Ellen knew the demands of balancing her career and family. She understood that her body needed to be in peak condition to keep pace.

Ellen discovered the benefits of lymphatic drainage—a therapy she found transformative. With each session, she felt her cells rejuvenating, her energy levels rising, and her immune system strengthening. Though there was nothing particularly wrong with her health, Ellen believed in preventive care. She came to my clinic regularly, not out of necessity, but to maintain her energy and ensure she stayed strong for her children and herself.

Ellen's visits became less frequent as life's demands grew. But one day, I received an unexpected call. "I've been training for a half marathon in Bali," Ellen explained, "but my legs have started cramping up and the pain is getting worse." Ellen was determined to finish her race, but her body seemed to rebel against her ambition.

I knew right away what was likely causing her discomfort. "Ellen," I said, "it sounds like your body is crying out for two things: salt and hydration. Without enough of either, your muscles can't function properly, especially under the strain of marathon training."

Ellen trusted my advice and scheduled a 90-minute lymphatic drainage session. We focused on rebalancing her system, addressing the cramping and fatigue that threatened to derail her race. The session worked wonders. By the time she left, the cramps had eased, and her energy levels had surged.

With renewed strength and vitality, Ellen continued her training, fully prepared for the challenge ahead. When race day arrived in Bali, she ran with a newfound power and resilience, quickly crossing the finish line.

Ellen's story is a testament to the incredible impact of under-standing and nurturing your body. It's not just about avoiding illness; it's about thriving, no matter the challenges life throws your way. And as Ellen proved, when you listen to your body and give it what it needs, there's no limit to what you can achieve.

86 CARMEL

Carmel walked into my clinic, a spirited 74-year-old with a quiet resilience that belied her years. She had recently undergone cutting-edge stem cell replacement therapy at one of Melbourne's premier hospitals—a revolutionary treatment that promised a lifeline for those battling terminal cancer. The results, they told her, were nothing short of miraculous. Her body, once riddled with disease, was now in a state of astonishing recovery.

But Carmel had one lingering concern. Despite the promising results, her legs had begun to swell—a troubling side effect that her doctors dismissed as inconsequential. Yet, the swelling weighed heavily on her mind and her spirit. Her once boundless energy had diminished, leaving her weary and uncertain.

In our first session together, I focused on alleviating her dis-comfort by addressing the swelling in her legs with gentle, targeted techniques. By the end of the session, the transformation was pro-found. Carmel's energy surged, her spirits lifted, and the swelling in her legs began to subside.

Over the next 12 months, Carmel continued her treatments with unwavering dedication. Each session restored more than just her physical strength; it rekindled a light within her, a vitality she feared had been lost forever. Slowly, as her body healed, she began to taper off the treatments, her visits becoming less frequent until, one day, she simply didn't return.

Her doctors were pleased with her progress at her monthly visits, and encouraged her to continue what she was doing.

Carmel's journey was one of quiet triumph, a testament to the resilience of the human spirit and the incredible potential of emerging therapies. Though it ended without a farewell, her story left a lasting imprint on my heart—a reminder that healing is as much about restoring hope as it is about curing the body. It shows that when we work together, everything is possible.

87   JORDY

The awakening of Jordy

Jordy was the epitome of health and vitality in her early twenties—fit, strong, and with boundless energy. Yet, despite her physical prowess, she began to experience a persistent pain in her legs that she simply couldn't understand. How could someone so young and seemingly invincible be suffering like this? The answer, as it turned out, lay deep within her.

During our first session, Jordy opened up about her life, and it became clear that the pain she was experiencing was more than just physical—it was the manifestation of years of unacknowledged stress and emotional turmoil. As the middle child in her family, Jordy had always felt a little overlooked, but the trustworthy source of her pain ran much more profound. Jordy was gay, and the weight of this identity, combined with societal expectations, had taken a toll on her body and soul.

She described the anxiety that had gripped her for years, the fear of rejection, and the dread of not being accepted by those she loved. Being true to herself felt like a risk she couldn't afford to take. The constant worry about how others would perceive her had created a storm of stress within her, and that stress was wreaking havoc on her body. It was as if her cells were being starved of oxygen, suffocating under the pressure of the secret she carried.

Over eight weeks, Jordy came to see me regularly. We delved deep into the conversations that mattered most, confronting the toxic beliefs she held about herself and her worth. With each session, we worked to cleanse her mind of the poisonous self-doubt that had festered for so long. As we cleared away the emotional debris, something remarkable happened—Jordy started to heal.

Oxygen is life, and as Jordy let go of her fears, it was as though she could finally breathe again. The pain in her legs subsided, replaced by a newfound sense of peace and self-acceptance. Jordy's journey was a testament to the power of healing, not just of the body but of the heart and mind. Jordy found the strength to embrace who she was—a vibrant, strong, and unapologetically authentic woman.

88   LILLIAN

Lillian's last fight

As the world emerged from the shadows of the Covid-19 pandemic, fear clung to the hearts of many, but none more so than Lillian.

In her sixties, Lillian was a fragile woman whose deep-seated terror of contracting the virus consumed her. She had been diagnosed with cancer, a cruel twist of fate that left her body swollen with lymphatic fluid, her right side bearing the brunt of this invisible enemy. The compression stockings she had been advised to wear provided little comfort, only adding to her discomfort and irritability. To the untrained eye, Lillian looked much older than her years, her face etched with the strain of survival. Lillian couldn't drive, so she relied on her friend for emotional and financial support. They attended my sessions together, splitting the cost to make it more affordable. Every fortnight, they would arrive at my clinic, Lillian's hope clinging to the belief that relief was within reach. But the fear—the relentless, suffocating fear—was an unyielding companion that no amount of treatment could entirely dispel.

Watching this beautiful soul wrestle with her pain and terror was heartbreaking. Her desperation was palpable, a quiet plea for the comfort that seemed always beyond her grasp. Despite the moments of temporary relief Lillian found in our sessions, Lillian's battle was an uphill one. The fear, the swelling, the cancer—it all weighed heavily on her, making every day a struggle. As time went on, the financial strain became too much. Lilian and her friend both loved coming and found a renewed energy after every session. The visits grew less frequent until, one day, they stopped altogether. The money had run out, and so had Lillian's strength to keep fighting alone. I never saw Lillian or her friend again; their story is a poignant reminder of the fragility of life and the battles that, despite our best efforts, we cannot always win. This is dedicated to Lillian, a woman of quiet strength whose story serves as a testament to the human spirit's enduring will to fight, even in the face of insurmountable odds. It is a story of hope, fear, and the tragic reality that sometimes, despite all the courage in the world, not all battles are meant to be won.

89 MICHELLE

The unseen wounds

Michelle's pain was palpable. She had a deep emotional wound that had festered for 23 years. She coped as best as she could with the weight of caring for her daughter, Laurna—a beautiful young woman trapped within the confines of her mind. Laurna could walk, but her speech was limited, and her comprehension of the world around her was fleeting. It was as if she was present in the body, but her spirit was unreachable. The strain of raising Laurna had eroded Michelle's 25-year marriage, leaving her isolated and burdened by a sense of guilt she could never escape.

Michelle's guilt was a constant companion, rooted in the belief that her choices during pregnancy had somehow condemned Laurna to a life of struggle. "If only I had said no," she would whisper, haunted by the notion that her daughter's challenges were a result of medical decisions made long ago. This self-blame gnawed at her, a relentless force that had manifested in physical pain. Her body was riddled with inflammation, the physical embodiment of 24 years of unresolved emotional turmoil.

Michelle had sought help from countless doctors, therapists, and healers, desperately trying to rid herself of the pain that seemed to have no end. But the problem was more profound than any medical treatment could reach. It was Michelle herself, clinging to the past, unable to forgive or release the guilt that bound her.

She came to me as a last resort, hoping for temporary relief. We began regular sessions, where I worked to ease the physical tension in her body, but the emotional scars ran too deep. Laurna also visited, and I gently massaged her tight muscles, doing what I could to offer comfort. Her body bore the marks of countless surgeries—rods in her back, ankles broken and re-screwed to help her walk again, and heavy medications that dulled her pain but not her spirit.

It was heartbreaking. I could provide some relief, but I knew the real healing had to come from within Michelle. She needed to let go of the past, to forgive herself, to release the guilt that had consumed her. But I could see it in her eyes—she wasn't ready, and perhaps she never would be.

And then, she was gone. One day, she simply stopped coming. I never saw her again. The pain, the guilt, the sadness—they were her burdens to bear, and Michelle had chosen to carry them alone. It was a chapter of her life Michelle couldn't close, and perhaps she felt she didn't deserve to.

Michelle's story stayed with me. A reminder of the invisible wounds we carry and the courage it takes to heal them. Some paths are too difficult to walk alone, and some battles are lost, not in the body, but in the heart.

90 MONIKA

The hidden cost of beauty

Monika was always beautiful. Her striking features, radiant smile, and vibrant personality turned heads wherever she went. But like many women today, Monika struggled with self-acceptance. The constant bombardment of unrealistic beauty standards and the pressure to look perfect made her feel inadequate. Despite her natural beauty, Monika needed to change her appearance to feel worthy of love and acceptance.

The decision to undergo cosmetic surgery wasn't made lightly. Monika opted for liposuction on her legs, a tummy tuck, and breast augmentation. She believed that by sculpting her body to fit societal ideals, she would finally achieve the confidence she so desperately craved. At just 27 years old, what Monika didn't realize was the hidden cost of these procedures—the long-term harm they would inflict on her body.

The surgeons painted a picture of quick fixes and instant gratification. Still, they failed to inform Monika of the complications that would arise later in life—the procedures left behind a trail of inflammation, scar tissue, and compromised circulation. The very surgeries meant to enhance her appearance ended up suffocating her body from the inside out. Scar tissue began to block oxygen from reaching her vital organs, leading to chronic pain and discomfort. Monika's journey didn't end with the surgery. Financial constraints meant she could only afford a few follow-up sessions before she had to return to her demanding job. As the days turned into weeks, her body began to harden, the pain became unbearable. Monika's once vibrant spirit dimmed as she grappled with the reality of her situation—her attempt to change her body had only made things worse.

The money Monika invested in these surgeries could have been used to embark on a 12-month journey of holistic transformation. This journey would have addressed the root of her emotional struggles and helped her learn to love herself just as she was. Instead, she was left with a body that no longer felt like her own and emotional scars that ran more profound than the physical ones.

Liposuction and similar procedures might promise quick results, but they often cost steeply in other ways. The removal of fat disrupts the delicate balance of the body, leading to an inflammatory response as it tries to heal. Scar tissue forms, not just on the surface but deep within, restricting the flow of oxygen and nutrients to vital areas. Over time, this can lead to a host of problems, from chronic pain to organ dysfunction.

Monika's story is a cautionary tale, a reminder that true beauty and self-love cannot be bought or surgically crafted. They must be nurtured from within. If she had been guided towards self-acceptance and natural healing, her story could have been about empowerment and transformation rather than pain and regret. At this moment, Monika is still struggling, her body a constant reminder of her choices. But there is hope. With proper support and a commitment to healing, Monika can begin to reverse the damage and rediscover her true self—a beautiful, worthy, and whole self, just as she is.

91   MICHAEL

Michael's miraculous recovery

Michael was in agony. The searing pain in his neck had become unbearable, so much so that even the slightest movement felt like torture. He could barely turn his head, and each day seemed worse than the last. Desperation finally drove him to pick up the phone and call me, hoping I could immediately squeeze him in for an appointment. When he arrived, I gently asked, "How long have you been struggling with this?"

"A couple of weeks now," he admitted, wincing as he spoke.

Why do people wait until the pain becomes unbearable before seeking help? It's a familiar story—ignoring the warning signs until the body screams for relief. But Michael was lucky. We caught it just in time.

During our session, I used my non-surgical techniques to address the root of his discomfort. When we were done, Michael could move his neck freely again. The relief was palpable, and he was astonished to feel 90% better after just one session. As the night wore on, the pain continued to fade, leaving him almost pain-free by morning.

This was yet another testament to the power of non-surgical healing. There was no invasive surgery, no dependence on pain medications—just the body's natural ability to heal when given the proper support. Michael's journey was a reminder that true healing is possible, even when all hope seems lost.

92   ANITA

Anita walked into my clinic seeking relief from relentless pain. But as I unraveled her story, it became clear that this pain was not just physical—it was rooted in something much more profound. Anita had been diagnosed with PTSD, a label that often comes with a heavy burden. It's far easier to pop a pill than to confront the emotional turmoil that lies beneath the surface. But I knew there was more to her pain than just a diagnosis. "Anita," I said gently, "you don't have Post-Traumatic Stress Disorder. What you're really struggling with is the belief that you're not good enough. You're trapped in a cycle of grief and sadness, and you can't see a way out."

She looked at me, stunned. "How did you know that?" Anita asked.

Years of intuition, awareness, and education have guided me to this moment. I've come to understand that physical symptoms are often the side effects of unresolved emotional trauma. Anita was carrying the heavy waste of her past, her energy depleted, her spirit exhausted. Every morning, she had to drag herself out of bed, the weight of her young children's needs only adding to her burden. Our first step was simple yet profound.

I guided Anita into deep relaxation, teaching her to breathe deeply and allow her body to release its tension. With each session of lymphatic drainage massage, we began to clear out the unwanted waste that had accumulated in her body—the physical manifestation of her emotional pain. The noise in her head, triggers, and destructive patterns began quieting. After just one session, Anita felt a shift within her. Anita couldn't quite articulate it, but her body had a newfound calmness, a lightness. At home, she noticed her actions were different, and her reactions were more measured. Could this be the turning point for her? I believe so, and not just for Anita but for anyone willing to confront the emotional roots of their physical pain.

Anita's journey demonstrates the power of addressing the whole person—body, mind, and spirit. Her story resonates with millions, offering hope that true healing is possible when we dare to look beyond the surface.

93   KADE

The lost soul of Kade

Kade stepped into my clinic, a shadow of the man he once was. At just 32, he looked a weary 52, his spirit crushed under the weight of a world that had betrayed him. The pandemic had snatched away his well-paying job, leaving him adrift, lost, and directionless. His mother had recommended my practice, desperate to save her son from the abyss he had fallen into. Kade's once-brilliant smile was now a painful reminder of his plight. His teeth were rotten, a clear sign of his body's inability to absorb protein, and the anger he harbored had drained the calcium from his teeth and jawline. This wasn't just a physical decay—it was the manifestation of the deep-seated rage he felt towards the world for robbing him of the life he had known. The world had stopped for him; in return, he had stopped caring.

Living with his aunt, Kade barely got by due to his dangerously low energy levels. He had become a prisoner of his mind, consumed by hatred for those he blamed for his shattered life. His savings were gone, spent on mere survival over the past four years, and his existence had become a tangled mess of despair and hopelessness. His mother watched helplessly, her grief deepening with each day as she saw her son slip further away. Kade's condition was dire. His lungs were lifeless, struggling to breathe, as if they were glued to his rib cage. He had been in survival mode for so long that he no longer recognized it. He needed more than just treatment; he needed to understand why his body was failing him. In a brief 15-minute conversation, I shared the knowledge and insight that could spark a change in him. It was like a light bulb flickered to life within him—a moment of clarity and hope he hadn't felt in years. This was the beginning of his journey to reclaim his life, to rise from the ashes of his anger and despair, and to find the strength to heal.

94   DOZICA

I had two sessions with Dozica who booked an appointment on a Friday afternoon, and by 5 pm she arrived, driven by her husband. As she sat down, her phone rang—it was her oncologist. She asked if she could take the call, and I nodded, sensing the weight of the conversation ahead. With the phone on loudspeaker, I listened as her doctor discussed her blood pressure, cautioning her about its dangerous levels.

As the doctor spoke, I could see the fear grow in Dozica's eyes. Her heart rate visibly increased as they discussed her blood pressure targets, the fear of an impending heart attack looming over her. Diagnosed with her second cancer just 12 months after having her ovaries and uterus removed, Dozica was about to turn 60, yet she looked like she had aged two decades overnight.

The doctor's reassurance that there was yet another pill for her if her blood pressure spiked felt hollow. I couldn't believe what I was hearing. Where had the wisdom of deep breathing and relaxation gone? Dozica was trapped in a stress response, agitated and overwhelmed by the way her health was being managed.

It took me just 15 minutes to calm her nerves and help her trust that she would be okay. I guided her to lie in the SOQI bed, the warmth enveloping her body. And then, something extraordinary happened. Her eyes rolled back momentarily before refocusing with an intensity I hadn't seen before.

At that moment, her innate intelligence reached out to me, and I began speaking to the core of her being. I told her that the anger and grief she carried were slowly killing her, that her past had haunted her for 50 years, and she could no longer push it away. Her body was crying out for unconditional love.

Tears welled up in her eyes as she asked, "How did you know?" She then revealed the deep wounds she had been carrying for decades. Her mother had died when she was just 16, followed by her brother four years later. The loss had been so devastating that all her dreams had died with them. Dozica, married, moved to Australia from Europe, and had twins, but never found happiness.

As she shared her story, Dozica took a deep breath, releasing years of pent-up emotion. The tension melted away, and for the first time in a long while, she relaxed, allowing herself to begin the journey of true healing.

When Dozica first walked into my clinic, the weight of her grief and recent cancer diagnosis seemed almost too much for her to bear. She carried an air of resignation as though the fight within her had dwindled to a mere flicker. The session I offered her was unlike anything she had ever experienced. It was foreign, strange, and perhaps even unsettling. But beneath her confusion was a glimmer of something that had been missing for far too long—compassion.

In that first encounter, I could see the depth of Dozica's sorrow and the layers of pain she had accumulated over the years. Yet, what she found most bewildering wasn't the treatment itself but the kindness she received. It was as if no-one had taken the time to understand her for a long time. Dozica had forgotten what it felt like to be heard, to have someone connect with her heart and soul without judgment or haste.

Dozica left the clinic that day, unsure what to make of it all. She was stepping into an unfamiliar world where unconditional love still existed. Despite her confusion, she re-booked for the following week. Perhaps some of her was curious, or she hoped this strange new world might offer her something she desperately needed.

The week that followed was filled with doctor's appointments and specialist consultations, a relentless parade of tests and results that only deepened her sense of exhaustion and hopelessness. Dozica was tired, lost in a maze of medical jargon and procedures, feeling as though her power had been stripped away, leaving her with little will to live.

When she returned for her next appointment, I greeted her with the same gentle understanding. I could see the weariness in her eyes, the quiet desperation she tried to hide. I offered her a loving, gentle lymphatic massage, focusing on her body and easing the fear that gripped her heart. As I worked, I could feel the tension slowly releasing, the barriers she had built around herself beginning to crumble.

When the session ended, Dozica thanked me for the massage and the understanding I had shown her. It was a small moment, but it was significant. In that simple expression of gratitude, I saw a spark of life returning to her, a hint that the will to live was still there, buried beneath layers of pain and fear.

Dozica had lost her power a long time ago, trapped in a cycle of tests and results that seemed to offer no escape. But in that quiet room, something began to shift with the soft words and gentle touch. The will to live, once nearly extinguished, was rekindled, if only just a little.

It is never too late to change. And for Dozica, the journey toward reclaiming her life had just begun.

95   HEIDI

Heidi's burden

Heidi was a 52-year-old woman carrying more than just extra weight—she bore the world's weight on her shoulders. Once vibrant, Heidi had fallen into a deep depression, a condition her doctors labeled and left her to navigate alone. With the label, they no longer needed to be responsible for her well-being. Now, Heidi lives with her elderly mother, surviving on a government pension she doesn't need, reinforcing her stagnant existence. Life moves along, but she remains isolated, far from the future she once envisioned.

Though she drives and participates in a singing group at her local church, the joy in Heidi's life is superficial. The pain she carries is far more profound, a heavy burden of unmet expectations and lost dreams. This was not how she pictured her life at 52. Her days are consumed by a vicious cycle of sugar-laden foods, chocolate binges, sleepless nights, and long, lonely days. She feels life has nothing to offer her anymore, and she, in turn, has nothing to strive for. It's a self-perpetuating program of "poor me," a cycle that's easy to fall into, but almost impossible to break free from.

Yet, something changed when Heidi decided to give me a chance. Her 81-year-old mother had been seeing me for her own health concerns, and had made remarkable progress—losing weight, reducing medications, and feeling revitalized. Inspired by her mother's transformation, Heidi hoped for the same.

After a few sessions with Heidi, I began to see her life patterns. Despite being attractive, she lacked drive in her personality. The spark that once defined her had dimmed, buried under years of emotional weight. Heidi's healing journey would not be easy, but I could see the potential for change—a glimmer of hope beneath the layers of despair. This was just the beginning of her path to reclaiming her life.

96   UNKNOWN

An inquiry from a lady with serious issues who found me on social media. She wrote me a letter asking for help.

Thank you, Michelle. My girlfriend Jacqui highly recommends you. Sadly, yes, I'm in the hospital, though thankful they gave me a few day passes to get some sleep at home. I am going back on Wednesday at 6 am for surgery, a bypass, an HP bypass to the right leg, and I will most likely lose my big toe. Many years ago, I had permanent birth control called ESSURE, which has caused a lot of damage, mainly due to high inflammation throughout the body. A class action went ahead this year against Bayer Pharmaceutical, and we are now waiting on the judge's ruling. Anyway, Jac thought you could help and suggested I contact you.

I'm sorry I haven't explained myself well. I am having surgery on Wednesday, pretty big surgery, 7 hours, apparently. They attempted going through my groin on Friday, but the central vein collapsed, typical me; nothing ever simple. They only let me leave for a few nights because I haven't slept since Thursday when I went to the hospital, plus I need to sort out a few other things, as I'll be in for just over two weeks, which will drive me nuts. Four days was bad enough. My foot has zero pulse in it, so my toe isn't the greatest to be honest. I thought I must have knocked and bruised it, which was back in July / August. I will catch up hopefully before Xmas.

Message from Michelle

One message can change everything in a world where true healing is elusive. Imagine this: "Your body is incredible. If only you allow it, it has the innate power to heal itself."

When Michelle, a world-renowned Lymphologist, shared these words, it wasn't just a passing comment—it was a lifeline. She knew that every cell in the body holds the potential for renewal, even in the face of overwhelming odds. She continued, "Your veins didn't collapse; they're filled with toxins and scar tissue. But that can be cleared with what I know. I've been taught by the very best, and everyone who comes to see me experiences a transformation in their health."

Michelle's confidence was palpable, a beacon of hope for those lost in the complexity of medical jargon and invasive procedures. "Going through surgery," she said, "will significantly impact your recovery and the repairing of your body. But remember, it's not the doctors or the surgeons who hold the key to your healing. It's you. I'm here if you need me."

Her words were more than just advice—they were an invitation to take control of one's health journey. The wisdom she imparted was born from years of experience and training under the most esteemed experts in the field of Lymphology.

Every person who crossed their path left not just healthier but with a renewed belief in the miraculous capabilities of their bodies.

"I wish you all the best," Michelle added with warmth. Remember, you may need lymphatic drainage to restore circulation to your body. I'm here to guide you whenever you're ready to begin this incredible journey."

Hi Michelle, I'm just letting you know the surgery went well, but sadly, they crushed my nerves, leaving me with zero feeling from the knee down, so I'm unable to walk without a frame. I'm hoping you can help with this.

She arrived at my clinic with her fragile frame, relying on a walker to move, her legs nearly lifeless from the burden of years of struggle. In just one session, we unlocked something profound within her— both legs began to regain strength, and the sensation returned to her limbs. She was astonished, her eyes wide with disbelief, yet I knew this was the body's natural capacity for healing at work. She walked out that day with renewed hope and a deep understanding that her body could restore itself.

But the weight of her emotional stress, accumulated over years, held her back. Despite the miraculous progress, she couldn't fully embrace the idea that such rapid healing was possible. Doubt crept in, and she returned to the doctors, seeking the familiar comfort of medication. The numbness soon returned, and sadly, she never returned to my clinic. That was the last time I saw her. Her story is a poignant reminder that healing is not just physical—it requires a shift in belief and the courage to trust in the body's innate ability to heal.

97   APHRODITE

The unspoken battle within Aphrodite

For over 20 years, Aphrodite had been chasing healing like a distant dream—one she couldn't quite reach. Born into a traditional Italian family, she was raised with one rule: be the good girl. And for her, that meant caring for everyone else first. But beneath the surface, her soul screamed for freedom. Aphrodite had carried the weight of her family's burdens for so long, always saying "yes" when every fiber of her being wanted to say "no."

Aphrodite had never admitted, even to herself, how deeply unfair her life had been. Her dreams, desires, and health were sacrificed on the altar of duty. The internal conflict between what she wanted and what she was conditioned to do was tearing her apart. She could feel it in her bones, muscles, and breath. The tension of living two lives—one for others and one longing to exist for herself—was killing her.

And like all silent wars, it eventually surfaced as illness.

Her chest felt weighed down by fear; her heart shattered from a love she couldn't extend to herself. She had a life that, from the outside, looked perfect—an adoring husband, a beautiful family, no apparent stresses. Yet her body was a battlefield, riddled with unexplained pain, fatigue, and exhaustion. Each passing year made it worse. Doctors were baffled, and offered no answers. Aphrodite felt trapped, watching her body deteriorate with no escape in sight.

When we spoke, I looked into her eyes and saw the truth her soul had been trying to tell her all along. Her pain wasn't just physical—it was emotional, born from years of denying herself. I explained that her suffering was the result of a lifetime of not standing up for herself. The fear she had been running from had been fuelling the inflammation that was consuming her body.

"You're terrified of ending up like your mother," I said, "even though the doctors tell you it's hereditary. That fear has been your shadow for far too long."

In just one 90-minute session, everything changed. Aphrodite left feeling lighter, more peaceful, and happier than she could ever remember. But the healing didn't stop there. Over the next few days, her body began releasing the poison it had held onto for years. She threw up dark brown and yellow fluid—decades of stuck inflammation finally finding its way out.

But like so many, life got in the way of her healing. Work crept back to the forefront, and her newfound clarity faded. I called Aphrodite a few weeks later to check in. Aphrodite admitted that while she had felt incredible after our session—less bloated, with energy soaring and her body working like it hadn't in years—something had shifted. She felt herself slipping back into old patterns.

"I need to come back and see you," she said, her voice tinged with exhaustion.

Aphrodite's story is one we all know too well: we put ourselves last, thinking it's noble and what we're supposed to do. But in the end, it's what makes us sick. It's what drains our spirit and our body. Healing begins when we decide, once and for all, to put ourselves first. Only then can we indeed be free.

98   JULIE

My story by Julie

Summer in February in Melbourne is typically hot and dry. The grass is burnt and brown with the heat, and the gum trees in the gardens of the suburban landscape omit their beautiful eucalyptus oils.

These are just some of the memories of when my nineteen-year-old self flicked through the booklets on nursing I had received from Alfred Hospital. The Alfred Hospital is situated in Melbourne's inner-city area of Prahran, and I was accepted into the nursing school.

I was waiting for the exciting and trepidant day I could start my training. I had worked in a banking center, processing cheques for twelve months. Although mind-numbing, it solidified that office work was not for me.

No other family members were nurse role models. In those days, it was more common for the older generation to make their careers out of being wives and mothers.

They started a careers guidance program in my final year of high school. I was encouraged to consider a career in kindergarten teaching, and my group was allocated a visit to a kindergarten and a small local hospital.

When the head nurse was called, the matron seemed to glow at the prospect of taking us high school students to the outside morgue.

Luckily, on that day, as she opened the door to the morgue,e there were no dead bodies present. It may have shifted any ideas of a nursing career away.

February 4th marked the beginning of a career in nursing and, later, midwifery that spanned four decades. Our student group, consisting of over eighty young women and two young men.

We all had an intense bond that still exists today. The support we offered each other was essential to our survival as new student nurses in a major public hospital. We worked together on different wards, gaining experience and maturity beyond our years.

Throughout my career, I have often been saddened by the plight of my fellow human beings. It wasn't just older people, but many young people as well. One particular memory was working in the Leukaemia ward. In those days, being diagnosed with leukemia was a death sentence. This was hard for me to deal with, as many of the patients were around my age. My life was so different from theirs, with the prospect of a career in nursing, youthful parties, and hope for the future.

However, a seed was being planted in my being. I was questioning why illness existed and why not everyone succumbed to disease.

A few books started coming my way, opening my eyes to the relationship between food, exercise, and environmental factors contributing to disease.

I was to experience some health challenges myself as I became older. At times, I didn't comprehend why these challenges came to me, as I was eating well, especially when I compared my lifestyle to that of others around me. I know now, with the wisdom of age, that I needed to learn lessons on a personal level to help others. I realized that not just food choices made up our health profile but other life choices. In my situation, I was dealing with shift work and long hours of stressful work with few breaks, which took its toll. At that stage of my life, I hadn't put together the effects of childhood trauma and the impact of negative emotional aspects on the body. That lesson was to come later.

One puzzle that I dealt with in my younger adult life was hypoglycemia, especially in the mornings. I worked with several naturopaths over this period, taking different potions and spending a lot of money to feel better. At around 30 years of age, I felt the call to start a family, only to be devastated by miscarriages.

My body finally accepted a pregnancy; a beautiful baby girl was my gift. As she snuggled into my arms, I felt joy beyond measure after so much sadness.

Life ticked along in my new role as a mother. Later, when I felt ready, I resumed my nursing/midwifery career part-time. When it came to wanting a second child, the health problems emerged, though they had never really gone away.

I was back on the merry-go-round looking for answers— more lessons to learn. The years passed with more miscarriages and no addition to our family.

I finally found a local naturopath named Eve. I walked into her room, sat down, and explained my situation. I will never forget her confident words: "Yes, we can have that baby you desire."

That day, my heart was full of hope, which had been lost. It was my lesson of how powerful words are; I believed her to be one hundred percent.

We went on a journey together, frustratingly identifying foods causing inflammation in my body and temporarily eliminating them. I also took a variety of herbal remedies, vitamin and mineral supplements, and angular therapeutic massage sessions.

One day, I was in Eve's waiting room when I picked up one of her books and started reading it. It was about liver cleanses. I chatted with Eve about it, and that became our next action plan. I gathered the ingredients and commenced the cleanse.

The difference I felt following the cleanse was terrific. Even though I functioned well enough before the cleanse, I realized what being healthy felt like days and months after.

Against many odds, I fell pregnant, and nine months later, precisely eight and a half years after my daughter's arrival, I snuggled up with a 4260-gram healthy baby boy.

During the first 20 weeks of the pregnancy, I learned a valuable lesson about mental health and how powerful the mind is over our health and well-being. I completely shut down from life and could barely function. I rode it out without any medical intervention, and like a switch, when I heard my son's heartbeat at the 20-week scan, the tears flowed with joy, and I was back to normal. I hadn't fully understood it at the time, but I had been protecting myself from another loss.

Working in maternity wards in the later years of my career, I gradually pieced together what I had learned during my training, and working in maternity wards was often not the best way for women to bring their babies into the world. This journey of discovery started in my early twenties when I was working in the field of District nursing. As the team's only midwife, I visited those who had had babies at the Queen Victoria Birth Centre. This was a new concept in midwifery care in Victoria, and the women would stay in the birth centre for only a short time before returning home. I don't know what words of wisdom I could give these fantastic women as newly trained midwives. However, the experience left me with respect for them and an interest in alternate ways.

During my two pregnancies, I was guided by a local practitioner and used Homeopathic remedies and Aromatherapy, unusual for those times.

In my continued career as a midwife in a private hospital, I observed many changes in care and protocols. Often, women felt powerless and in fear. Increasing rates of interventions such as inductions, epidurals, and cesarean sections were observed.

During those years, I was present with women who had completed natural childbirth classes. I was amazed at the difference between these women, their general calmness, and their confidence in having and nurturing their babies.

When I spoke to these women after they had their babies, one course that came to my attention was Hypnobirthing. I learned a lot, and I studied until I was right. A seed had been planted.

A few years later, I completed the Hypnobirthing Australia course and began taking classes whenever possible. What a world this course opened for me. I had to abandon many of my commonly held beliefs, which I had learned through my traditional midwifery training. I loved it all, and it aligned well with my faith in the human body's power when given the best environment to function as we were designed.

During the busy years of working and caring for my family, I felt a strong calling to find spiritual meaning in my life. This led me on many adventures, including travels overseas. On one trip to South America, I met and became friends with Jenny. Jenny recently changed her career path and became an Emotional Freedom Techniques (EFT) Trainer. EFT, also known as Tapping, has many clinical studies behind it.

Of course, I also completed this course, and along with the Hypnobirthing course, I now realize the power of our thoughts and beliefs. Opportunity came my way when I was offered the Lactation Consultant position at the hospital where I was working. I said yes, as I had had enough of working in the birth suite. I studied hard, completed the International Board-Certified Lactation Consultant (IBCLC) qualification, and built up the clinic within the hospital. For the first time, I felt the sense of independence I craved. I thoroughly enjoyed interacting with the mothers, babies, and families as I guided them through their breastfeeding journey.

Times were changing, and I was incredibly saddened when I had to walk away from what I loved doing in October 2021 when the government mandates and hospital policies no longer aligned with my views on health or the knowledge I gained as I did my diligent research.

I was lost for a while after this, as retiring from the workforce, ending my career, and being unable to help people were not on my radar.

A chance phone call from a friend asking me if I would be interested in attending a presentation by Dr Darryl Wolfe started a new journey in a completely different direction. Dr Wolfe's presentation aligned with my understanding of health and wellness, and I was inspired to look for something new.

Michelle organized the evening, and at the end, my friend and I introduced ourselves to her. After this meeting, Michelle gave a community presentation at a hills community group. I learned more about her work with the lymphatic system, the energy bed (SOQI bed), and the E-Power belt. Subsequently, I booked in to take her Lymphology Australia course and added lymphatic drainage massage to my modalities.

I started working with a few clients and loved the work as clients responded well to the lymphatic drainage. It is an excellent opportunity to share my health and wellness knowledge with anyone open to this.

And there was more.

Michelle also introduced me to Wolfe's non-surgical bodywork, and I booked appointments for some health issues I was experiencing.

I was impressed by how it made a difference for Michelle's practice, me, and other clients. When Michelle informed me that Dr Wolfe's son, Sage, was coming to Australia to teach non-surgical bodywork, I booked my place in the course and headed up to Coffs Harbour to complete the course in August 2024, with some good friends.

That brings us to the present. As I edit and complete my story, I can feel a fundamental shift in the world's energy.

My client booking numbers have suddenly increased for all the different modalities I offer. I have my first non-surgical bodywork client booked for next week.

I am very grateful for the work I am doing. I know I can guide others to heal themselves when they are ready, and that motivates me to get up every day with lots of energy and a spring in my step.

99   UNKNOWN

She entered my clinic, a small, frightened figure trembling like a tiny mouse. Her eyes, glazed and distant, rolled back into her head, betraying a life of pain and unresolved anguish. She was only 60, but the weight of her emotions made her seem much older.

As I took a deep breath, the room seemed to fill with an unspoken energy. I felt it instantly—the deep, festering wounds of hatred and grief she had carried since childhood, now rotting her from within. "Your emotional world is in ruins," I gently told her, "hanging on to these dark feelings is poisoning you."

Tears welled in her eyes, a mixture of relief and disbelief washing over her. "How did you know that?" she asked, her voice trembling.

I smiled softly, feeling the presence of her innate spirit speaking to me. "Your spirit communicated with me," I replied, "I feel everything—every hurt, every hope—and I receive messages that I share with those who need to hear them."

100   SOPHIE

My journey began the minute I was born. I came into the world in a body that did not want to work correctly, into a miserable family and unstable home. It took me most of my life to understand that all of this had been the instigation of the myriad of health issues that I was to suffer.

I have spent 55 years seeking an answer to my increasing health concerns. Beginning with digestive problems and food intolerances (dreaming of living on only air and water), gynecological issues, insomnia, skin conditions, debilitating headaches, fibromyalgia, circulation problems, cellulite, weight gain and loss, bloating, and pain. And the list goes on. One issue morphed into the next, and it was difficult to know what needed to be treated most, as each wanted to compete and take priority.

I have sought the advice of countless medical professionals, tried all types of complementary and alternative therapies, spent tens of thousands of dollars, and, most importantly, expended so much energy looking for a reason and remedy. My health ruled my life. Sometimes, it was every minute of every day. It never went away. It was never out of my mind. Then, strangely, my health would improve and I would feel excellent and on top of the world. But I never knew exactly why.

When my body returned to what it always did, I struggled to return to when it was good—always searching for answers, trying new things, and never giving up. One step forward, one step back, plateauing. The desperation to find an answer is all-consuming. I never knew what it felt like to live normally. But I knew that I should be able to.

After moving to The Dandenongs, I looked for a local therapist. I was tired of running around Melbourne to get to my various appointments. Indeed, there was someone up here who could help me.

Michelle is a breath of fresh air. She takes a very different approach to lymphatic drainage than I had experienced before, and she uses a very different infrared sauna, where I can move into the SOQI bed. Her extensive training and knowledge put her far above anyone I had seen in lymphatic drainage therapy.

Michelle is interested in caring for my health, treating me, and educating me to help me understand why my body is doing what it's doing.

At each non-surgical session, I tell Michelle what treatment I would like. She listens to what I say, think, and feel, although she just knows what my body needs. I can feel the effects as I am being treated. I do not need to wait until the end of the session to feel calm, light, even, stable, and free, which I always do. Throughout the session, I am given information and education, and I leave knowing more about myself and my health.

I would love to finish the session quickly in the SOQI bed. As soon as it is switched on, I feel the energy in my body. I feel like I am coming to life, and there is an instant calmness.

There is no upselling, no telling me what I need, no unnecessary treatments, no booking me into appointments before I leave. The care is for me and my health, not in sales and marketing, which, unfortunately, you can fall victim to when you are on your quest for healing and health.

After a few months of treatment by Michelle, I know I am permanently on the path to health. I feel fabulous, do not have to constantly think about what is wrong and how to fix it. I am calm and free, and my mind is clear. It's a strange feeling: not being constantly clouded and stressed to find an answer I'm looking for. I am no longer in the wilderness of confusion.

Thank you, Michelle. Thank you for being a part of my journey to health, which is now much shorter than I ever thought it could be.

A new dawn in healing

You may wonder how so many people with such diverse and complex health challenges have achieved such remarkable results so quickly. The answer lies in delivering education, a deep understanding of their issues' root causes, and the lymphatic system's power. Imagine a world where chronic illnesses aren't just managed, but they are truly healed. Where the body's innate intelligence is honored and harnessed for real, lasting recovery.

For decades, I've witnessed firsthand how the lymphatic system and non-surgical approaches can transform lives. My name is Michelle Richardson. As a Lymphologist, I've guided countless individuals back to health, not through invasive surgeries or endless medications but through a profound understanding of the body's natural healing mechanisms.

I have shared stories with you of real people who faced real challenges. These aren't just tales of overcoming adversity; they are testaments to the power of cellular regeneration, the strength of the human spirit, and the efficacy of non-surgical methods. These stories show that addressing the root cause of illness, rather than merely treating symptoms, opens the door to true healing.

Imagine a mother of five, crippled by pain after multiple surgeries, finding hope and strength to heal without further invasive procedures. Picture a man whose life was burdened by the weight of heartache for 72 years, finally discovering health and returning to his homeland renewed. Consider the countless others who have come to me with stories of despair and left with renewed hope, vitality, and a new lease on life.

These aren't isolated incidents—they are part of a more significant movement, a new era in healthcare in which we thrive rather than survive together; we can embrace this groundbreaking approach to healing and cellular regeneration, which makes a difference and changes everything.

By understanding and addressing the root causes of illness, we can pioneer a new era of health and well-being. This isn't just about our generation; it's about our children, our loved ones, and the future of our world. Let's take charge of our health, explore non-surgical solutions that genuinely heal, and make a lasting impact on the lives of those we care about.

The end... but really, a beginning

This is not the end of our journey—it's merely the beginning. The stories shared here are just a glimpse of what is possible when we look beyond conventional medicine and embrace our bodies' full potential for healing. The path forward is clear: it's time to revolutionize how we approach health, educate, inspire, and heal— not just ourselves but the world around us.

Real stories, impact, and healing are our legacy, our gift to the next generation. Let's embrace it together.

Now is the time to take your health and education to the next level. Imagine a world where illness, sickness, and disease no longer define our lives. That vision is within reach and starts with empowering yourself with the knowledge and tools to heal and thrive.

To embark on this life-changing journey, I invite you to connect with Professor Karl West, Dr Darrell Wolfe or myself. Together we offer revolutionary, life-saving education designed to transform your health and the health of everyone you touch.

Join us in creating a new era in healthcare—one where healing is natural, comprehensive, and accessible to all.

Recommendations

Mandy Smith

Inside Out Whole Healing Hub

Retreat 500 acres of natural bush

New South Wales Australia

Your body's capacity to heal is greater than anyone has permitted
you to believe

Call Mandy on 0429 408 296

References

These resources provide a comprehensive overview of the lymphatic system, its significance in health, and ongoing research in the field. Here are five references that provide credible information about the lymphatic system:

1. "The Lymphatic System in Health and Disease" by J. A. Zawieja and M. T. Scallan This book offers a detailed exploration of lymphatic biology, including its structure, function, and role in diseases.

2. Guyton and Hall's Textbook of Medical Physiology is a comprehensive textbook on physiology. It includes an excellent section on the lymphatic system and its functions in maintaining fluid balance and immunity.

3. "The Lymphatic System: A Clinical Perspective, by David W. Stoller and Michael D. Flynn, is a clinically oriented resource focusing on the lymphatic system's anatomy, imaging, and pathophysiology.

4. "Lymphatic Research and Biology" (Journal) This peer-reviewed journal publishes cutting-edge research on lymphatic system biology, disorders, and innovative treatments

5. Samuel C. West was a proponent of the lymphatic system's role in health and developed educational materials on the subject. Here are some references related to his work and general resources on the lymphatic system: The Golden Seven Plus One: A self-help book by Samuel C. West focusing on the lymphatic system and methods to maintain its health

Index

For more information and to be part of this groundbreaking movement, Let's reshape the future of health together.

Contact Prof Karl West

https://speedhealing.com/

Contact Michelle Lymphologist

https://www.lymphologyaustralia.com/

Contact Dr. Darrell Wolfe

https://docofdetox.com/

www.ingramcontent.com/pod-product-compliance
Lightning Source LLC
Chambersburg PA
CBHW051243020426
42333CB00025B/3030